BODY PAIN
AND
PAIN RELIEF

DR. ABU HENA MAHBOOB
MBBS, FCPS (SURGERY), MS (ORTHOPEDICS AND TRAUMATOLOGY)
ORTHOPEDIC SURGEON

Copyright © 2022 by Dr. Abu Hena Mahboob and MedHelp Centre Inc.

All rights reserved.

Edited by Dorelle Hinton

Illustrations by Daniela

Cover Design by Trisha Fuentes.

Published in Canada

No part of this book may be reproduced in any form or by any electronic or mechanical means, including information storage and retrieval systems, without written permission from the author, except for the use of brief quotations in a book review.

Krishnadayal Chakrabarty
assistant teacher
Ram Kishore High School, Muktagacha,
Mymensingh, Bangladesh.

You opened the doors to the world for me and inspired me to be the best that I could be. Thank you, sir, for being the best teacher I ever had.

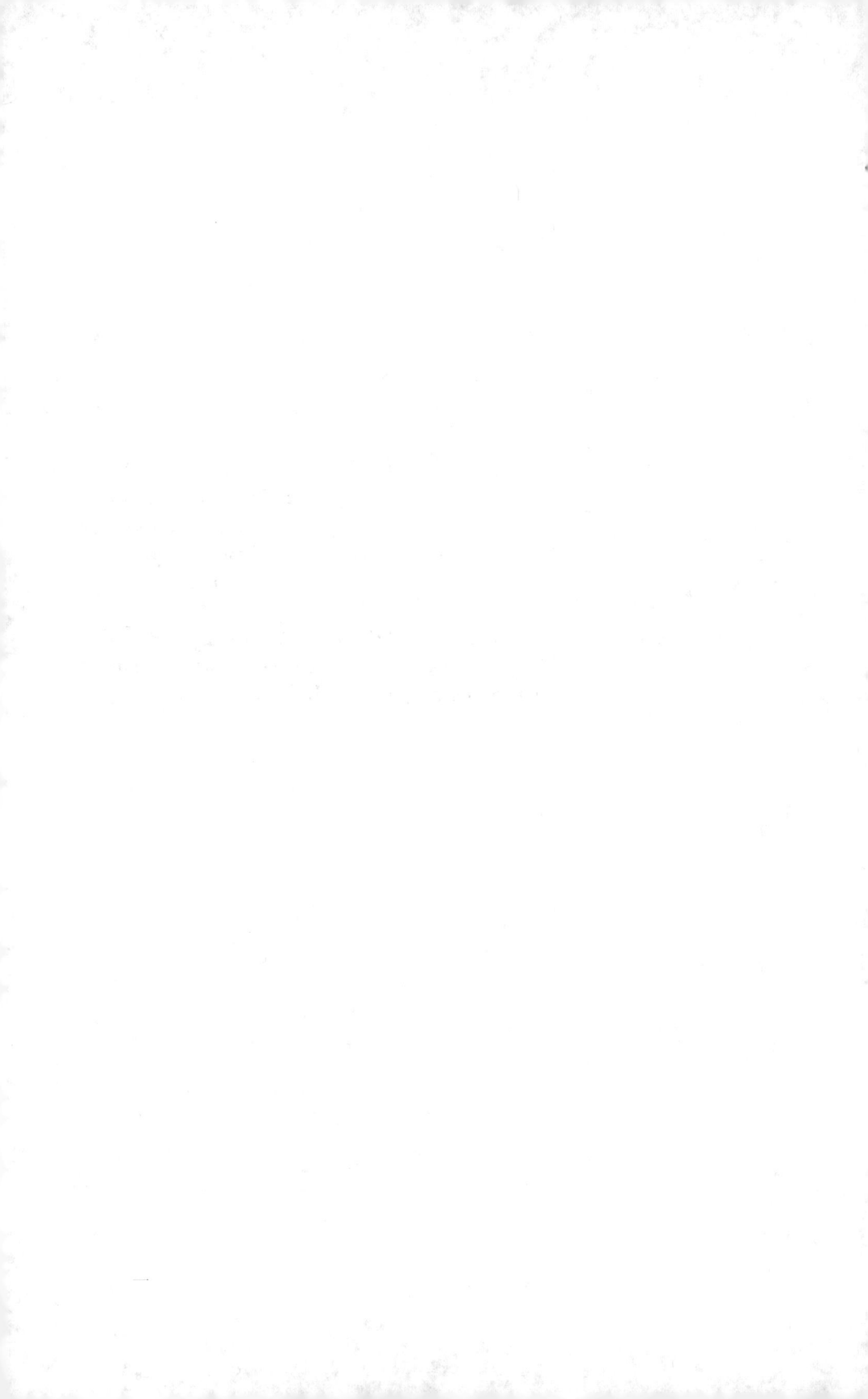

Contents

About the Author ix

Preface xi

Pain of Abdomen and Pelvis 1
Pain in the Anus 23
Pain in the Testes 29
Body Pains in Seniors 33
Bone Infection and Pain 47
Bone Tumor and Body Pain 49
Chest Pain 51
Diabetes and Body Pain 77
Ear Pain (Earache) 87
Eye Pain 91
Nose Pain 99
Fibromyalgia 103
Gout and Body Pain 107
Hand Pain 111
Finger Pain 127
Foot and Heel Pain 135
Frozen Shoulder 145
Headache 149
Hip Joint Pain 165
Joint Infection and Pain 169
Kidney and Renal Pain 171
Liver Pain 179
Knee Pain 185
Low Back Pain 191
Menopause and Body Pain 201
Menstrual Cramp 207
Ovulation Pain 211

Muscle Pain	213
Neck Pain	215
Osteoarthritis (OA) and Joint Pain	225
Ankylosing Spondylitis (AS)	231
Osteoporosis and Body Pain	235
Prostate Enlargement and Pelvic Pain	243
Elbow Pain	247
Pregnancy and Body Pain	253
Rheumatoid Arthritis (RA)	265
Shoulder Pain	273
Wrist Pain	279
Appendices	*287*
Glossary	*309*
References	*311*

Nothing begins, and nothing ends,

That is not paid with moan;

For we are born in other's pain,

And perish in our own. [Daisy]

–Francis Thompson (1859-1907)

Each patient is an unique entity.
Their perception of pain is also different and should be treated as such.

About the Author

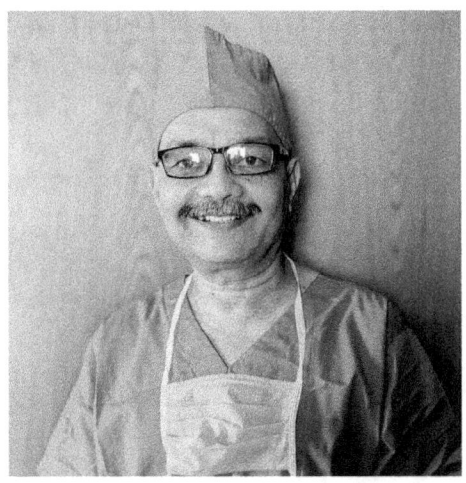

Dr. Abu Hena Mahboob

Dr. Abu Hena Mahboob, an experienced and renowned orthopaedic surgeon in Bangladesh, was born at his maternal grandfather's house located in a remote village called Chakbandi under the district of Sherpur.

He received his early education at Municipal Primary School and Ramkishor High School at Muktagachha, and at Anandamohan College in Mymensingh. Later he earned his bachelor's degree in medicine (MBBS) from Sylhet Medical College, and went on to obtain a fellowship in surgery (FCPS) from Bangladesh College of Physicians and Surgeons, and a master's in orthopaedic surgery (MS) from National Institute of Traumatology and Orthopaedic Rehabilitation, University of Dhaka. At a later stage he completed his fellowship in Arthroplasty at Delhi Institute of Orthopaedics and Traumatology (DITO) and Indraprastha Apollo Hospital in Delhi. He was also awarded registration from Medical Council of India.

Dr. Mahboob had been engaged in teaching surgery and orthopaedic surgery in different medical colleges in Bangladesh for a period of about three decades. He possesses immense experience and exceptional skills in the art of surgery which, apart from being his profession, is also a passion with him.

His loving wife Sultana Morjina is a gynaecologist and resides in Canada while his only son Mahboob Hasan Mehdee is a student and an entrepreneur, based in Canada.

Dr. Abu Hena Mahboob is used to living his life in his own style. He is deeply fond of music and travel. In his free time, or freeing himself from work, he often goes on tours around the country or abroad.

His mind is always ablaze with scientific curiosity, reasoning and questioning.

Preface

Pain is the voice of the body.

As an orthopedic surgeon, I have been working with different kinds of physical pain for nearly 35 years. Over the course of my career, I have realized that there are some common pains that are suffered by a vast majority of people, but many patients are sadly incapable of expressing and explaining those to healthcare professionals. In this book, I have tried to explain the nature of such pains so that patients can understand those better and pinpoint their complaints to physicians. This book also features some home remedies which can help combat certain forms of pain in their earlier stages through preventive and alleviative measures. I have mentioned the possible complications not to panic the patients but to make them aware of those so that they can follow the proper course of action in time.

If this book helps you understand your pains better and encourages you to take appropriate measures to ease your problems, I shall consider my efforts successful.

Author

Pain of Abdomen and Pelvis

Happy Tummy Happy Life

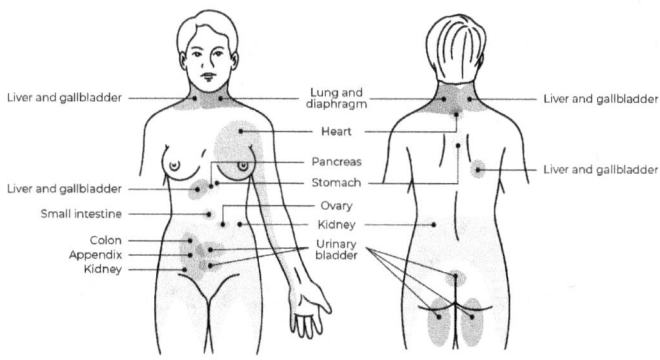

Pain from internal organs is referred to the skin.

The abdomen is also called the 'belly' or 'tummy' and is the part of the body between the chest and the pelvis. The abdominal cavity contains several organs and is also known as a temple of surprise.

Abdominal pain is the pain that originates from the organs of abdominal cavity. Almost everyone has pain in their abdomen at some point in life. Abdominal pain can be described as crampy, achy, dull, intermittent, or sharp. Most of time, this pain does not signify a serious condition. The degree or seriousness of abdominal pain does not always reflect the seriousness of the condition causing the pain. Sometimes a very bad abdominal pain occurs due to a relatively mild condition, where your safety is not at risk. However, a very serious condition may present as a mild pain or without any pain at all.

Infection, inflammation, or other diseases that affect the organs in the abdomen and pelvis can cause abdominal pain.

The major organs located in the abdomen and pelvis are:
- the stomach, small and large intestine.
- the appendix, a part of the large intestine.
- the peritoneum, a thin covering of the abdominal cavity and abdominal organs.
- the gallbladder and biliary system, which includes the *liver, pancreas,* and *spleen.*
- the urinary system, which includes :
    o two *kidneys*, organs which form urine.
    o the *urinary bladder*, an organ which reserves urine.
    o the *ureter,* a tube connecting the kidney and urinary bladder, and
    o the *urethra,* a tube connecting the urinary bladder to the exterior.
- large blood vessels and
- the internal genital organs :
    o Female : *Ovaries, uterus, fallopian tubes,* and *peritoneal folds.*
    o Male : *prostate* and *seminal vesicles.*

Bacterial, viral, and parasitic infections, different types of chronic and acute inflammations, tumors, and obstruction or blockage of tubes affect the organs of the abdomen and may cause significant pain in the abdomen and/or pelvic region of the body.

There are different types of pain that are experienced in the abdomen.

Generalized abdominal pain
Generalized abdominal pain is described as being felt in more than half of the belly. If generalized abdominal pain becomes more severe, it may be deemed due to a blockage of the intestine.

Generalized abdominal pain is more typical for:
- Inflammation of the stomach lining.
- Indigestion, stomach gas, or gastroenteritis.
- Generalized inflammation of the peritoneum.
- Inflammation of the pancreas.
- Psychogenic pain, and/or
- Pain due to metabolic disturbances.

Localized abdominal pain.
Localized abdominal pain is felt in only one area of the abdomen. It is more likely to be a sign of a problem in a single organ, such as the appendics, gallbladder, or stomach. The most common cause of localized pain is stomach ulcer.

Cramp-like pain.
Cramp-like pain starts suddenly and is intermittent in character. It arises especially from the abdominal and pelvic viscera. This type of pain may be accompanied by gas, bloating or diarrhea, constipation and/or flatulence. In most cases, cramp-like pain is not serious. Signs of a more serious include cramp-like pain that occurs more often, lasts more than 24 hours, or occurs with a fever. Cramp-like pain may also occur in the skeletal muscles.

Colicky pain.
Colicky pain comes in waves and occurs due to spasm in any hollow or tubular soft organ, such as the colon, gallbladder or urinary tract. This type of pain very often starts and ends suddenly and is often severe. Urinary stones, and gallbladder stones are common causes of this type of abdominal pain.

Upper abdomen.
The upper abdomen is the region of the abdomen above the level of belly button (umbilicus).

Causes of upper abdominal pain in both sexes :

- *Gallbladder*: Stone. Infection. Inflammation. Tumor.
- *Kidney*: Stone. Infection. Inflammation. Tumor.
- *Liver*: Inflammation (hepatitis). Abscess in the liver. Tumor.
- *Stomach* :
    - Reflux of acid from stomach to esophagus (the tube connecting the oral cavity to stomach).
    - Gastritis or- Inflammation of stomach lining.
    - Stomach ulcer.
    - Dyspepsia or indigestion.
    - Gastroparesis - Delayed emptying of stomach.
    - Tumors.
- *Spleen* : Enlarged spleen. Rupture of spleen.
- *Pancreas* : Inflammation (pancreatitis) and obstruction in the duct of pancreas by stone or tumor

- *Intestine:*
  - Irritable bowel syndrome. Constipation.
  - Obstruction of intestine. Tumor.
- *Lung*: Pneumonia.

Lower abdomen

The lower abdomen and pelvic region is the area between the level of the belly button (umbilicus) and the groin. The pelvic cavity is bound by the bones of the pelvis. The roof of the pelvis is the pelvic inlet and is continuous with the lower abdominal cavity. The lower boundary of the pelvis is the pelvic floor.

Causes of lower abdominal and pelvic pain in *males*:

- *Intestine*: Irritable bowel. Constipation. Obstruction.
- *Appendics.*
  - Appendicitis: Inflammation of the appendix.
  - Tumor.
- *Ureter*: Stone in the ureter.
- *Urinary bladder.*
  - Infection and inflammation (cystitis).
  - stone in the urinary bladder. tumor.
- *Prostate and seminal vesicles.*
  - Prostatitis: Infection and inflammation of prostate. Pus in the prostate.
  - Enlarged prostate. Tumors of prostate.
  - Sexually transmitted infections in prostate and seminal vesicles.
- *Internal and external urethra.*
  - Urethritis: Sexually transmitted urethral infection.
  - Stone in the urethra. Urethral constriction.
- Chronic pelvic pain syndrome.
- Chronic peritoneal adhesions.

Causes of lower abdominal and pelvic pain in *females*: Generally in women, pelvic pain may be a sign of menstrual cramps and/or pain due to ovulation.

- *Intestine*: Irritable bowel. Constipation. Intestinal obstruction. Tumor.
- *Appendics*:
  - Appendicitis: Infection and inflammation of the appendics. Tumor in appendics.

- *Ureter*: Stone. Tumor. Infection.
- *Urinary bladder.*
  - Cystitis: Infection of the urinary bladder.
  - Stone. Tumor.
- *Urethra.*
  - Infection (urethritis). Stone. Tumor.
  - Urethral constriction.
- *Uterus, fallopian tubes, ovaries, and peritoneal folds*
  - Tumors of the uterus (fibroid, cancers)
  - Pelvic inflammatory disease (PID).
  - Sexually transmitted infections.
  - Ovulation pain. Menstrual cramps.
  - Ectopic Pregnancy : pregnancy outside the uterus. Lost pregnancy.
  - Muscle spasm in the pelvic floor.
  - Urinary tract infection.
  - Torsion of the ovary.
  - Ovarian tumor. Cysts of ovary.
- Chronic pelvic pain syndrome.
- Chronic peritoneal adhesions.

Causes of severe abdominal and pelvic pain:

- Rupture of a tubed organ like the intestine, appendix, fallopian tube, large blood vessels.
- Gall stone diseases.
- Stones in the urinary system.
- Infection of the urinary and gallbladder system.

Causes of lower back and pelvic pain:

Pain related to

- Kidney, ureter, and urinary bladder.
- Genital organs.
- Pelvic part of the intestine.

Features of most common abdominal and pelvic pains :

Appendicitis
Infection and Inflammation of the appendics.

The appendics is a narrow finger-shaped pouch that projects out from the large intestine on the lower right side of abdomen. Appendicitis is an infection and inflammation of the appendics. Appendicitis is a surgical emergency. If it is suspected, immediate hospitalization is mandatory.

Features of appendicitis:

- Sudden pain in the right side of the lower abdomen.
- Sudden pain that starts around the umbilicus and shifts to the lower right abdomen.
- Pain worsens upon walking, coughing or other movements involving the abdomen.
- Nausea and vomiting.
- Low-grade fever.
- Abdominal bloating and flatulence.

As soon as appendicitis is suspected, the patient should be taken to the emergency room. This is a surgical emergency.

Stomach ulcer

The stomach is a muscular organ located on the left side of the upper abdomen. The stomach receives food from the esophagus. Esophagus connects the mouth to the stomach. To digest food, the stomach secretes strong acid and enzymes. Normally, the stomach has several self defence mechanisms, including the mucus-bicardbonate barrier, to protect the stomach against both the acid and enzymes. If, for any reason, this protection is broken, the acid and enzyme actions will cause a stomach ulcer.

Features of stomach ulcer:

- Burning stomach pain or burning sensation in the chest.
- Pain is felt in the upper middle part of the abdomen , just below the breastbone (sternum).
- Pain is burning or gnawing.
- Feeling of fullness, bloating, or belching.
- Acid reflux in the mouth.
- Nausea and vomiting.
- Not wanting to eat because of the pain.
- Pain is relieved by taking anti-ulcerant drugs.
- Pain may worsen between meals and at night.

Home remedies for *stomach ulcer* pain:

- Control of mental and physical stress through physical exercise, yoga, and meditation.
- Warm bath.
- Drinking plenty of water eliminates the acid from the stomach and gives soothing effects.
- Lemon water for indigestion : The alkaline effect of lemon helps in soothing the excess acidity in the stomach.
- Anti-acidity suspensions neutralizes acids in the stomach.
- Whole grains and a high-fiber, low-fat diet : Fiber helps to absorb stomach acid and helps to stop the symptoms of acid reflux.
- Green vegetables including Cabbage, cucumber, broccoli, and kale.
- Ginger, garlic, turmeric, cloves, and cinnamon act as anti-inflammatory agent.
- Cumin seeds : reduces hyper acidity, gaseous distention of the abdomen, and pain.
- Banana helps to reduce irritation by forming a coating over the ulcer and combatting discomfort. Due to its high fiber content, banana also absorbs stomach acid.
- Apples, cherries, red grapes, and other colored fruits.
- Mint leaves : Mint contains menthol that helps to make stomach calm and reduce indigestion problems.
- Aloe vera juice reduces acid reflux.
- Honey, amla.
- Yogurt : probiotics in yogurt help to normalize bowel function and soothes stomach discomfort.
- Cold plain water, lemon tea, green tea, unsweetened milk.
- Nuts and seeds.

In stomach ulcers, *avoid* :

- Overeating.
- Deep fried foods.
- Smoking. Alcohol. Coffee.
- Carbonated beverages. Sugar.
- Hot and spicy foods. Chilis and hot peppers.
- High salt containing foods. Processed foods.

Not every food acts in the same way for every person. So, keeping track of which foods make your symptoms worse and avoiding these foods will give more relief.

When to seek medical advice with a stomach ulcer:

- A sudden sharp pain in upper abdomen and the condition steadily worsens.
- Severe nausea and vomiting.
- Vomiting of blood : Blood may appear as bright red, dark brown, or grainy in appearance like coffee grounds.
- Stool may appear dark and tar-like.
- Constant abdominal pain and feeling of bloating.
- Severe heart burn and appetite loss.

Gastroenteritis

Gastroenteritis is a short-term illness caused by infection and inflammation of the lining of the stomach and intestinal tract. It is also called the 'stomach flu'.

Features of gastroenteritis:

- Sudden onset of loose, non-bloody, watery stool.
- Nausea and vomiting.
- Abdominal pain or cramps.
- Mild to severe dehydration.
- Mild fever. Lack of energy.
- Muscle aches, or headaches.

Dehydration : Dehydration occurs when more fluid is lost from the body than the amount of fluid taken. Due to lack of water and other fluids, body cannot carry out its normal functions.

Features of dehydration:

- Dry mouth, tongue, and skin.
- Feeling very thirsty.
- Less frequent urination.
- Dark-colored urine.
- Feeling tired and weak.
- Muscle cramps.
- Lightheadedness on standing.
- Confusion.

Home remedies for mild gastroenteritis:

- Proper hydration of the body is a must. Plenty of fluid intake like plain water, oral rehydration solution and soup.
- Foods or drinks with potassium : fruit juice, bananas etc.
- Fluid should be taken regularly throughout the day, especially after each bout of diarrhea.
- Age-appropriate small meals are better. Eating should be in small amounts and done often and include some salty food.
- Ginger tea and drink, chamomile drink, sips of plain water.
- Let the stomach to settle and calm.
- Solid food should be stopped for a few hours.
- Sufficient physical and mental rest.

  Avoid:
  o Spicy and fried foods.
  o Caffeine. Alcohol.
  o Raw and dried vegetables and fruits.
  o Excess fiber-containing food.
  o Whole grain breads, brown rice and cereals.
  o Milk and milk products like cheese, yogurt.

Medications should be taken as per physician advice. Hospitalization may be required if bowel motion is not controlled and features of dehydration develop.

Constipation

Constipation is a decrease in a person's normal frequency of defecation and is accompanied by difficult or incomplete passage of hard and/or dry stool. Constipation occurs most often due to changes in diet or routine of food intake, or due to inadequate intake of fiber in meal.

Features of constipation ::

- A decrease in a person's normal frequency of defecation.
- Passing fewer than 3 stools in a week.
- Pain in the anus after defecation.
- Stomach ache or cramps.
- Feeling of bloating and nausea.
- Stool is dry, lumpy, hard, difficult and/or painful to pass.
- Straining is required to have a bowel movement.

- Feeling as though there is a blockage in the bowel that prevents bowel movements and cannot be emptied completely from the bowels.
- Bowel movement needs the help of a finger to remove stool from the bowel.
- Sometimes fresh bleeding through the anus may occur after the end of passing stool.

Home remedies for constipation:

- Drinking plenty of water.
- Diet should contain more fiber, especially soluble, non-fermentable fiber e.g, Psyllium husk, beans, lentils, oat, peas, apples with skin, chia seeds, flaxseeds, skins of many fruits and vegetables.
- Physical exercise like walking, swimming, cycling, jogging.
- Senna, a herbal laxative.
- Drinking coffee as it stimulates the muscles in the gut.
- Probiotic foods e.g. yogurt, saukraut, kimchi, which contain live, beneficial bacteria that naturally occur in the gut.
- OTC laxatives : bisacodyl, senna, sennosides, castor oil, aloe, magnesium citrate etc.
- Prebiotic foods : garlic, onions, bananas, chickpea, leeks, chicory etc.
- Dairy products may be avoided as they can cause constipation.

If home treatment does not relieve symptoms, consultation with a physician is required.

Irritable bowel syndrome (IBS)

Irritable bowel syndrome is a common disorder that affects the large intestine. It is a chronic condition and requires a long term management. Everyone experiences irritable bowel differently, with symptoms varying from one time point to the next.

Features of irritable bowel:

- Abdominal cramping or bloating, usually in the lower belly, related to a bowel movement.
- Increased gas or mucus in the stool.
- Changes in the number of bowel movements.

- Altered bowel habits, including chronic or recurrent diarrhea, constipation, or both, either mixed or in alteration.
- Rectal bleeding.
- Food intolerance.
- Feelings of stress, depression, or anxiety which can also make irritable bowel worse.
- Weight loss. Fever. Anemia.

Home remedies for irritable bowel:

- Problem foods should be identified and avoided.
- Foods that trigger symptoms should be eliminated.
- Plenty of fluid intake is advised.
- Meals should be taken at regular times. No meals should be skipped and must be taken at about the same time each day to help to regulate the bowel function.
- Regular physical exercise like walking, jogging, running, swimming, cycling etc. are continued.
- Avoiding Stress. Enough sleep.
- High-fiber foods are advised, like brown rice, oatmeal, whole wheat, green peas, beans, apple with skin, turnip green.
- Avoid high-gas foods like carbonated and alcoholic beverages and coffee.

Some people with irritable bowl are sensitive to certain foods like lactose and fructose. These are found in certain grains, vegetables, fruits and dairy products and should be avoided.

Foods high in lactose (should be avoided):

- Milk and milk products.
- Yogurt, cheese, icecream.
- Cakes, cookies, pies.
- Pastries, cream and cheese filled pastries.
- Pudding, chocolate, custard, ice milk.
- Caramels.

Foods low in lactose, which are relatively better:

- Breads and baked goods.
- Milk chocolate.
- Breakfast cereals.

- Instant soups. Cereal bars.
- Salad dressings. Sauces.

Lactose-free foods and drinks (,these which are the best):

- Soya yogurt and cheeses.
- Almond and hazel nut milk, yogurt and cheese.
- Coconut-based yogurts and cheese.
- Oat milk. Rice milk.
- Dairy-free foods.

Foods with high fructose should be avoided with IBS. They are:

- Apple and apple juice.;
- Dry figs.; Grapes.;
- Watermelon.;
- Honey and molasses.;
- Palm and coconut sugar.;
- Caramel.;
- Peas.; Asparagus.;
- Invertd sugar.

Lower fructose foods, which are relatively better:

- Bananas.; Carrots.; Avocados.;
- Green beans.; Lettuce.

When to seek medical advice in IBS:

- Symptoms that develop after the age of 50.
- Sudden severe abdominal pain and extreme changes in IBS symptoms.
- Symptoms persisting for a long time.
- Appearance of blood and mucus in stool.
- Development of new symptoms.
- Unintentional weight loss.
- Blood in stool and severe anemia.
- Severe cramping in the abdomen and activities of daily life are hampered.
- OTC medications do not relieve symptoms.
- Severe diarrhea or constipation or problems in urinating.
- Strong-smelling and foul-smelling gas.
- Repeated vomiting.
- Fever along with symptoms of IBS.

Immediate medical advice should be sought in the following conditions:
- Sudden severe abdominal pain.
- Blood in the stool.
- Family history of IBS and appearance of symptoms.
- Joint, skin or eye discomfort.
- Sudden severe diarrhea.
- Pain in the abdomen that is getting progressively worse.
- Significant loss of appetite.
- Sudden weight loss, or dizziness.
- Symptoms that occur only at night and cause sleep disturbance.

Inflammatory bowel disease (IBD)

IBD comprises two conditions : Crohn's disease and ulcerative colitis. IBD is a long term inflammation of the gastrointestinal tract resulting in tissue damage to the gut.

Features of IBD:
- It is a persistent or long-lasting i.e. chronic disease.
- Symptoms vary depending on the severity of inflammation and which part of intestinal tract is involved.
- Symptoms may range from mild to severe and have periods of active illness followed by a period of remission.
- Abdominal pain and cramping.
- Severe urgency to have a bowel movement.
- Diarrhea and blood in the stool.
- Fever.
- Loss of appetite and weight loss.
- Anemia and feeling of fatigue.

Extra-intestinal features of IB:
- Joint pain, with the joints of spine being mainly affected.
- Eye inflammation.
- Mouth and skin ulcers.
- Liver inflammation and jaundice.

Home remedies for inflammatory bowel disease:
- Frequent small meals are advised.
- Drink plenty of liquids like water or electrolyte beverages.

- Dairy products should be limited.
- Calcium, vitamin D, and other vitamin supplements.
- Probiotics like yogurt is beneficial.
- Prebiotics : stimulate growth of healthy bacteria in the gut. They are (garlic, onion, leeks, bananas, asparagus, dandelion greens etc).
- Aloe vera : acts as a strong anti-inflammatory agent.
- Regular physical exercises : walking, jogging, running, cycling, swimming etc.
- Yoga to reduce stress.
- A low-fiber diet is beneficial.
  - Cooked vegetables : spinach, pumpkin, eggplant, skinless potatoes, beans, squash, carrots, beets etc.
  - Refined grains.
  - Yogurt. Poultry and eggs.
  - Ripe fruits : bananas, papyas, watermelon, plums, peaches etc.
- Reducing the consumption of fatty foods.
- Foods with strong anti-inflammatory effects : turmeric (curcumin), ashwagandha, Psyllium seeds.
- Omega-3 fatty acid supplements.
- Fish oils, pineapple, and camels' milk are beneficial.
- Soft and liquid diet.

When to seek medical advice in IBD:

- Repeated abdominal pain and diarrhea.
- High and prolonged fever.
- Excessive bleeding with stool.
- Unintentional loss of weight.
- Repeated vomiting and diarrhea leading to dehydration.
- Severe abdominal pain accompanied by repeated vomiting and excessive bloating.
- Features of abdominal obstruction:
  - Vomiting.
  - Abdominal pain.
  - Absence of bowel movements.
  - Distention of abdomen.
- Painful joints.
- Changes in vision.
- Low blood pressure and fast heart rate.

Inflammation of the pancreas

The pancreas is an organ situated in the abdomen behind the stomach. It functions as a gland, secreting mainly (99%) digestive enzymes. A small part of the gland (1%) secretes some essential and life saving hormones.

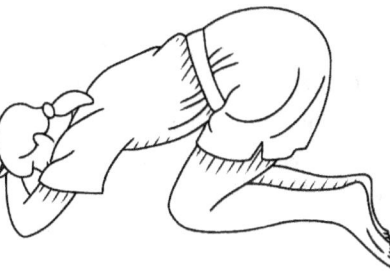

Pain relieving position for pain in pancreas

Causes of inflammation of pancreas:

- Gallbladder stones blocking the pancreas tube.
- Infection and inflammation of the pancreas (pancreatitis).
- Injury in the abdomen.
- Obesity. Alcoholism.

Features of inflammation of the pancreas:

- Upper abdominal pain, which may be constant or that returns.
- Pain may radiate to the back.
- Pain feels worse after eating.
- Leaning forward or assuming a fetal position (curling-up) may help to lessen the pain slightly. It is also called as 'knee-chest position' on right or left side.
- Nausea and vomiting.
- Increased pain on touching the abdomen.
- Oily and smelly stool and where the stool floats on water.

- Diarrhea for long duration.
- Weight loss.
- Features of diabetes.see page:
- Fever. Rapid pulse.

When to seek medical advice:

It is best to seek medical advice as early as inflammation of the pancreas is suspected.

Inflammation of the peritoneum (peritonitis)

The peritoneum is a vast thin membrane that covers the whole of the inner wall of the abdominal cavity as well as the organs within the abdominal cavity. The peritoneum also supports the abdominal and pelvic organs and serve as a supporting channel for blood vessels, lymphatic vessels, and nerves.

Causes of inflammation of peritoneum:

- Perforation in the stomach, intestine or any hollow organ within the abdominal cavity.
- Infection and inflammation of any organ of abdomen.
- An abdominal trauma.
- Rupture of any abdominal organ.
- Unknown causes.

Features of inflammation of the peritoneum:

- Abdominal pain, loss of appetite.
- Fever.
- Pain on touching the abdominal wall.
- Feeling of fullness and distention of abdomen.
- Bloating.
- Nausea, vomiting, and diarrhea.
- Inability to pass stool or gas, on occasion.

When to seek medical advice:

It is best to seek medical advice as early as peritonitis is suspected.

> *Kidney or renal pain: page*
> *Menstrual cramp : page*

Ovulation pain : page
Tumor of uterus (fibroid)

Uterine fibroids are an extremely common condition. They are solid tumors that develop in the uterine wall and are made of smooth muscle cells and fibrous tissues. Fibroids may appear as single tumor or in a group that vary in size and in shape. Each tumor may be as small as a seed or as large as a melon. Fibroids are not cancerous and do not increase the risk for uterine cancer. The exact cause of fibroids is not known.

Risk factors of fibroid formation:

- Genetic factors as fibroids may run in families.
- Prolonged exposure to estrogen hormone.
- Obesity.
- Diets high in animal protein.
- High blood pressure.

Features of uterine fibroids:

- Pelvic and lower abdominal pain.
- Heavy menstrual bleeding. Longer menstrual periods.
- Bleeding between menstrual periods.
- Infertility.
- Lower backache.
- Pain during sexual intercourse.
- Complications during pregnancy :
    o Recurrent pain in abdomen and pelvis.
    o Recurrent vaginal bleeding.
    o Spontaneous miscarriage. Preterm labor.
    o Fetal malpresentation.
    o Placental failure.
    o Increased postpartum hemorrhage.
- *Bladder* symptoms :
    o Increased frequency of micturition.
    o Difficulty in micturation and feeling of incomplete micturaition.
- *Bowel* symptoms:
    o Constipation.

When to seek medical advice:

- Heavy menstrual bleeding.
- Persistent lower abdominal and pelvic pain.
- Heaviness in the lower abdomen.
- Recurrent miscarriage.
- Features of anemia : such as pale skin, fatigue, weakness, chest pain, cold hands and feet.

Pelvic inflammatory disease (PID)

Pelvic inflammatory disease (PID) is an infection of one or more of the female upper reproductive organs, which include the uterus, uterine (fallopian) tubes and ovaries.

Causes of PID:

- Unprotected sex and/or multiple sexual partners causing the entry of different types of infecting organisms into the uterus. Organisms may also enter into the uterus during menstruation, child birth, miscarriage, or abortion.
- Insertion of IUD.
- Douching regularly.

Features of PID:

- Mild to severe lower abdominal and pelvic pain.
- Fever.
- Heavy vaginal discharge of unpleasant odor.
- Abnormal uterine bleeding.
- Pain during intercourse.
- Painful and difficult urination.

When to seek medical advice:

- Severe pain in the lower abdomen.
- Foul smelling vaginal discharge.
- Nausea and vomiting.
- High fever.

Chronic pelvic pain

Chronic pelvic pain is the pain in the pelvic area that lasts for 6 months or more. Chronic pelvic pain may come and go, may remain constant, or it may follow a regular menstrual cycle. Chronic pelvic pain can range from a dull ache to a sharp pain.

Causes of chronic pelvic pain:

- Musculoskeletal diseases like diseases of the bones, joints, ligaments and other soft tissues in the pelvic region.
- Muscular tension in the pelvic floor muscles.
- Inflammations affecting the joints of pelvic region.
- Chronic pelvic inflammatory diseases.
- Pain may arise from digestive organs :
  o Chronic constipation.
  o Irritable bowel.
  o Food intolerance.
  o Appendix problems.
- Pain may arise from urinary and genital organs:
  o Infection in urinary bladder.
  o Prostate problems.
- Pain may be caused by irritation of the nerves in the pelvis.

Features of chronic pelvic pain:

- Pain is felt in the lower abdomen and pelvic area.
- Pelvic pain may be associated with low back pain.
- Pain is severe and steady.
- Pain may be dull aching, sharp and cramping.
- Sometimes the pain is intermittent, and it comes and goes.
- Feeling of heaviness in the pelvis.
- Pain during sexual intercourse.
- Pain during bowel movement and urination.
- Pain while sitting for long period of time.

Home remedies for pelvic pain:

It is best to seek medical advice for pelvic pain.

BODY PAIN AND PAIN RELIEF

If it is not serious, some measures may be tried at home, like:

- OTC drugs : Ibuprofen, Naproxen, Acetaminophen.
- If constipation is the cause, see page :
- Relaxation and muscle stretching exercises.
- Deep breathing exercises. chart
- Sufficient sleep.
- Use of hot water bottles/heating pads.
- Smoking and alcohol cessation.
- Vitamin D, E, and magnesium supplements.

When to seek medical advice:

- Sudden, severe pelvic and lower abdominal pain.
- Pain is associated with vaginal bleeding.
- Pain disrupts activities of daily life.
- Severe nausea and dizziness.
- Pain is associated with fever.
- Pain is getting worse over time.

Psychogenic pain

Psychogenic pain is a physical pain that is caused, increased or prolonged by mental, emotional or behavioral factors. A psychogenic basis has often been assumed as the cause in diagnosis of recurrent abdominal pain when clinical examination and laboratory tests show no organic or medical reasons for the pain. This type of pain is an unpleasant sensory and emotional experience associated with actual or potential tissue damage. Many people report pain in the absence of tissue damage or any likely obvious cause . Usually this happens for psychological reasons. A common psychogenic pain is stomach pain. This type of pain is induced by social rejection, grief, broken heart, or other such traumatic events.

When to seek medical advice:

It is better to seek medical advice as early as pyschogenic pain is suspected.

Metabolic disturbances causing abdominal pain

In metabolic disturbances, there are some derangements in the blood biochemistry. Common conditions include very high blood sugar level in diabetes, and increased and decreased activities of some hormone producing glands.

In uncontrolled diabetes, metabolic disturbance will cause generalized abdominal pain, and pain may be accompanied by nausea, vomiting and dehydration. Getting control of diabetes and functions of other endocrine glands will relieve the abnormalities and pain. Abdominal pain may also occur due to other unknown causes.

When to seek medical advice:

- Sudden and severe abdominal or pelvic pain.
- Fever.
- Dull abdominal pain that lasts for more than one week.
- Pain that worsens, becoming more severe or occuring more frequently.
- Loss of appetite and gradual weight loss.
- Blood mixed with stool (*'Tarry stool'*)
- Vomitus contains blood.
- Persistent nausea, vomiting and dehydration.
- Yellowish discoloration of the skin or eyes.
- Severe pain on touching the abdominal wall.
- Abdominal distention.
- Abdominal pain with respiratory distress.
- Inability to have a bowel movement.

When to seek medical advice for pelvic pain due to unknown causes:

- Severe pelvic pain.
- Pain changes its intensity or frequency.
- Gradually increasing pain.
- Pain is accompanied by :
    o Fever. Nausea and vomiting.
    o Blood in the urine or stool.
    o Foul-smelling urine. Cloudy urine.
    o Weight loss.
- Pain does not go away, despite home care efforts.
- Pain goes away but returns.

Pain in the Anus

The anus is the outlet of the digestive tract that opens to the exterior. The anal canal, measuring about 4 centimeters, is the tube at the end of the large intestine and is the end of digestive tract. The anal canal opens into the anus.

Anal pain is a common complaint and is the pain that occurs within the anal canal and around the anal opening. Almost all causes of anal pain are not life threatening. The anal canal and the surrounding area, the perianal region are richly supplied with pain nerve endings, and the pain in this area can be very severe. Anal pain can be highly distressing, but it is often just the result of a minor and highly treatable problem. Many conditions cause anal pain as well as bleeding through the anus. The conditions are usually more frightening than serious.

Causes of anal pain:

- *Tear* in the anal canal wall due to passage of hard stool or other causes. This is called *anal fissure*.
- Severe *constipation* causing pain after defecation.
- Prolonged or chronic *diarrhea*.
- *Levator ani syndrome*: Spasm in the muscles that surround the anus.
- *Perianal abscess*: Pus in the deep tissue around the anus and anal canal.
- *Hemorrhoids*: Swollen and inflamed veins around the anal canal.
- *Fistula*: Abnormal channel between the anal canal and the skin near the anus.
- *Infection* in the anus by bacteria or viruses including fungal infections or sexually transmitted infections.
- Inflammatory diseases of the intestinal tract like i.e. Crohn's disease.
- Anal itching and pain due to *pruritus ani*.
- *Proctalgia fugax*: Recurrent pain in the anus due to rectal muscle spasm.
- *Cancer*, *ulcers* and *inflammation* in the anal canal.
- *Trauma* to the anus, anal sex.
- *Coccydynia*: Repeated trauma and inflammation around the tailbone.
- *Skin diseases* around the anus e.g,. wart.

Common causes of anal pain and their features.

Anal fissure

An anal fissure is a longitudinal tear in the wall of the anus.

Features of anal fissure:

- History of long-term constipation and hard stool.
- Severe sharp pain during passage of stool.
- Gnawing or burning pain in the anus.
- Bleeding from the anus.
- Bright red blood on stool and bleeding after defecation.
- A visible crack may be found in the skin around the anus.
- A small lump or skin tag may be present in the skin near the anal fissure.

Home remedies and prevention of anal fissure:

- Must practice regular bowel habit.:
- Stool should be kept soft by adding more fiber to diet and drinking plenty of water. Foods with high fibre include: broccoli, cabbage, celery, cucumber, lettuce, spinach, watermelon, tomato, fruits with skin, whole grains, beans, peas, and seeds.
- After each bowel movement, a warm sitz bath is helpful.

Sitz bath or hip bath: It is a warm, shallow bath that is done by soaking the perineum in a tub of warm water, two or three times a day. Perineum is the space between the anus and the vulva or scrotum.

Benefits of sitz bath:

  - It cleanses the perineum.
  - Can promote healing of an anal fissure.
  - Relief pain and itching in the anus and genital area.
- OTC stool softeners: milk of magnesia, dulcolax etc.
- Use of local anesthetic ointments to decrease pain.
- Skin around the anus should be kept clean.
- Regular physical exercises such as walking and running are beneficial. A sedentary lifestyle enhances the onset of constipation.
- Never delay going to the toilet when a defecation urge is sensed.

When to seek medical advice:

- Severe pain in the anus after each bowel movement.
- Bright red blood on the surface of the stool.
- Bowel movements are so painful that going to toilet is avoided by the patient.
- Severe constipation and anal pain with fever.

Hemorrhoid

Hemorrhoids are dilated and swollen veins in the anusveins. They, are also called as piles. They are one type of varicose vein.

Features of hemorrhoids:

- Pain and discomfort in and around the anus.
- Painful bowel movements.
- Swelling around the anus.
- Repeated bleeding through the anus.
- A hard lump near the anus which is painful to touch.
- Leakage of fecal matter.

Home remedies and preventions:

- Must practice regular bowel habits.
- High-fiber diet: vegetables, fruits with skin, whole grains.
- Plenty of water intake.
- OTC pain relievers: hemorrhoid cream or suppositories.
- Regular warm sitz baths.
- Cold compress to the anus.
- Physical activities should be continued.
- Sitting for long period of time should be avoided.
- Wearing of loose fitting, breathable, cotton clothing and underwear helps in wound healing, reduces irritation and prevents the worsening of inflammation.

When to seek medical advice:

- Repeated bleeding through the anus during and after bowel movements.
- Home treatment does not improve the condition.
- Severe anal pain and bleeding.
- Sudden changes in bowel habits which may signifying a more serious condition.

Anal itching and pain

Anal itching and pain are common conditions. Sometimes there is an intense itching around the anus that is accompanied by a strong urge to scratch resulting in soreness and pain.

Common causes of anal itching and pain:

- Yeast infections. Pinworms.
- Sexually transmitted diseases (STD).
- Anal fissure.
- Allergic reactions. Dermatitis.
- Hemorrhoids. Anal tumors.
- Spicy foods. Long term diarrhea.
- Associated with some systemic diseases
    o Diabetes.
    o Long term Liver and Kidney diseases.
    o Anemia. Cancer in the body.
- Anxiety and depression.
- Fecal incontinence causing skin irritation.

Features of anal itching:

- Intense anal itching.
- Redness and soreness around the anus.
- Redness and burning sensation.
- Blister formation around the anus.
- Dry cracked skin.

Home remedies and prevention:

- Anus and surrounding skin should be kept clean.
- Plain water cleansing is best.
- Warm sitz-bath may help.
- Scratching should be avoided.
- Regular bowel movements are maintained.
- Stool should be kept soft to firm.
- A high fiber-containing diet should be taken.
- Wearing of loose fitting, breathable, cotton clothing and underwear helps in wound healing, reducing irritation and preventing the worsening of inflammation.

When to seek medical advice:

- Severe and persistent anal itching.
- Skin rash around the anus.
- Leakage of stool.
- Discharge from the anus.
- A lump in or around the anus.
- Itching disturbs sleep and activities of daily life.
- Recurrent bleeding through the anus.
- Itching accompanied by weight loss, fever, or night sweats.
- Itching affecting whole body.
- Itching & pain does not improve with home-care measures.

Pain in the Testes

The testes are male reproductive organs located in the scrotum. Scrotum is a loose bag skin on the exterior of the body. The main function of scrotum is to maintain a cooler temperature compared to the internal body temperature for the testes. On average, the temperature of the scrotum is 3°- 5° centigrade cooler than the normal body temperature. Normally, there are two testes. They develop within the abdominal cavity and enter the scrotum in the later stages of development in the utero.

Pain in the testis may be caused by minor conditions like minor trauma, or there may be more serious causes of pain in the testis. So, it is better alwaysst to always pay attention to pain in the testis.

Common causes of pain in the testis:
- Trauma to the testis.
- Infection and inflammation of tissues around testes.
- Orchitis : Infection of the testis.
- Twisted testis. Tumor in testis.
- Renal stones (ureter/urinary bladder stones).
- Infection and inflammation of the prostate.
- Urinary tract infections, STD.

Features of some common conditions of testis:

Trauma to the testis
Trauma to the testis is not uncommon and may be minor, where no specific treatment is required. However, sometimes the trauma is serious and can damage the testis.

Home remedies for minor testicular trauma:

- Scrotal support.
- Ice compression applied to the area.
- OTC pain relievers.

Medical advice is required if the patient suffer from any of the following symptoms after a trauma.

- Severe pain in the testis that lasts longer than an hour.
- Swelling in the testis or scrotum following a trauma.
- Bruising of the scrotum.
- Nausea, vomiting, or fever following trauma to the testes.
- Penetrating injury to the scrotum or testis.

Orchitis:

Infection and inflammation in the testis.

Features of orchitis:

- Severe pain in the scrotum.
- Swelling of the scrotum and testis.
- Severe pain on touching the scrotum.
- Fever and chills. Nausea and vomiting.
- Painful urination.
- Feeling of fatigue.

As soon as infection in the testis is suspected, immediate medical attention is necessary.

Torsion/rotation of testis

Torsion of testis occurs when a testis is rotated and the cord which suspends the testis becomes twisted. As a result, blood flow to the testis is blocked and gradually the testis dies.

Features of torsion:

- Most commonly occurs between the ages 12 and 20 years, but it can occur at any age.
- Sudden, severe pain in the scrotum.
- Swelling of the scrotum.
- Fever and chills. Nausea and vomiting.

- Lower abdominal pain.
- The affected testis climbs at a higher level as compared to its pair.

Torsion of testis usually requires emergency surgical intervention. If treated quickly, the testis can usually be saved.

Tumor of testis

Testicular tumor is not so common. Any palpable lump and hardness of a lump must be evaluated by a physician as soon as possible. Hard lump in the testis that is painless to touch should get special attention.

Features of testicular tumor:

- Painless lump in the testis is common and early feature.
- Pain, swelling and Feeling of heaviness in the scrotum.
- A dull ache may be present in the groin.
- Typical testicular sensation may be lost.
- A general feeling of malase or unexplained fatigue.
- Fever, s weating.
- Mild chest pain and shortness of breath.

As soon as a testicular tumor is suspected, medical advice must be sought.

How can you maintain good testicular health ?

The testes must be kept cool and should be 3°- 5° centigrade less than the normal body temperature. As such, repeated and prolonged hot baths should be avoided as well as using a laptop on the lap, as the laptop can increase the temperature of testes.

Other tips for good testicular health include:

- Wearing loose-fitting cotton underwear.
- Regular physical exercise.
- Regular sexual activity and regular ejaculation.
- Quitting smoking.
- Preventing testicular injury.
- Maintenance of good body hygiene.

BODY PAIN AND PAIN RELIEF

Foods that are beneficial for healthy testes:

- D-aspartic acid suppliements.
    - Animal proteins, white meat.
    - Peas and beans.
    - Nuts. Lentils.
- Foods rich in anti-oxidants. See page:
- Food supplements :
    - Fish oils. Calcium. Zinc.
    - Vitamin C, D and E.
    - Ginger.
- Avocados, Carrots, Tomatoes, Spinach, Dark chocolate.
- Whole grain cereals, Legumes. Fresh fruits and vegetables

Body Pains in Seniors

'Age is a matter of mind, if you don't mind, it doesn't matter'.

–Mark Twain.

Pain is the voice of the body. As injurious agents begin to damage the areas of body parts, the body gives signals by producing pain to protect the body from these injurious agents. As the life span becomes longer, more and different types of pain develop. The assessment and treatment of repeated onset of pain in the body of older adults (over age 65) are special challenges for healthcare workers.

The body is a mechanical system and the ageing process causes the breakdown of this mechanical system after many uses over many years. The effects of aging are caused by progressive damage to cells and body systems over time. Once the cells wear out, they can no longer function correctly.

Pain in the elderly is common but not an inevitable part of aging. Without any obvious cause, there may be body pain in the elderly. Older age group patients has lower pain tolerance. Always body pains are not the signs of weakness or loss of self dependence. Bed rest is not always the best remedy for long term pain. Medications are not always required to relieve pains. Pain generally relieves by home remedies.

There are many functional systems in the body. One is bone, muscle and joint (musculo-skeletal) system, which is more or less visible from outside and other systems are concealed in different body cavities which are not obviously seen.

Musculo-skeletal system includes the following main structures:
- Bones (i.e, the skeleton).
- Muscles attached to the bones.
- Tissues that support and bind organs together: Cartilage, tendons, ligaments, joints etc.

The primary functions of musculoskeletal system include:

- Body support.
- Allowing motion between different parts of the body.
- Facilitation of movements and locomotion. Protecting the internal organs.
- Storage of minerals and fats.
- Hematopoiesis: production and development of blood cells.

Changes occur with aging in all the components of the musculoskeletal system. These changes will cause symptoms which are characteristic of the aging process.

Effects of long-term musculoskeletal pain:

- Disinterest in ambulation and activities of daily life.
- Fear to move or complete personal activities of daily life.
- Reduced participation in household activities.
- Functional dependence on other members of the family.
- Feeling of weakness in the hands, feet and legs.
- Gradual increase in disability.
- Abnormal postures in walking, sitting and lying.
- Changes in behavior and reaction to different emotional matters like joy, sorrow, and grief.
- Sleep disturbances.
- Preferring social isolation.
- Mental anxiety and depression.

About 85% of older adults suffer from pain in somewhere in the body. Common pains include:

- Back pain.
- Pain due to body stiffness.
- Joint pain: Hip, knee, neck, ankle, shoulder, wrist, hand, foot, fingers. Headache.
- Osteoporosis and body pain.
- Fibromyalgia (chronic pain illness)
- Muscle pain (polymyalgia rheumatica).

Back pain
Majority of people experience pain in lower back in their life.

Common causes of back pain:

- Aging.
- Leading a sedentary lifestyle.
- Overweight.
- Poor food habits and lifestyle.
- Poor body posture in sitting, standing, walking and sleeping.

With age, water content in the spine decreases, making the spine stiff and less flexible, resulting in pain during movement and activities. Aging is also a major factor in causing the narrowing of the lumbar spinal nerve passages, infection, tumors and osteoporotic (porus bone) vertebral fractures. Muscle strains, ligament sprains, inflammation of vertebral joints, compression fractures of vertebral bodies due to trauma or osteoporosis, osteoarthritis (loss of joint cartilage and inflammation of bones and soft tissues associated with joints) and rheumatoid arthritis (inflammation of joints due to some unknown causes) are also responsible for back pain in older adults.

Detailed features of back pain: page

Home remedies for back pain:

- Heat applied to the lower back region. Benefits, see chart.
- Limited bed rest. *'Motion is lotion'* in back pain.
- Remaining active. As the saying goes, 'motion is lotion' for back pain. Continuing physical activity when pain is mild to moderate can help to alleviate pain.
- Massage to relax the aching muscles. Benefits, see chart.
- Stretching and strengthening exercises of the back muscles according to advice from the physiotherapists.
- Use of firm (not too hard nor too soft) mattresses. Benefits, chart.
- OTC pain relievers: Ibuprofen, Naproxen, Acetaminophen.

Prevention of back pain in older adults:

A healthy body posture must be practiced while standing, walking, sitting and sleeping. As such, it is best to sleep on either left or right lateral side with bent knees and a pillow in between the knees. It is also adviced that older adults maintain a healthy body weight, a healthy and balanced diet, and remaining physically active.

Prolonged bed rest can actually make lower back pain worse. Walking is the best exercise and can be continued if pain is mild or moderate.

Regular physical exercise helps to keep the muscles of the back and abdomen strong and flexible, reducing stress on the back itself. Other advices are:

- Prolonged static posture must be avoided. One minute of walking in every hour is beneficial.
- Adequate sleep. Benefits: chart.
- Stretching exercises for limb and back muscles.
- Swimming in warm pool. Benefits: chart.
- First kneel before bend forward.
- Avoid lifting heavy objects. Rules to lift heavy objects: Page
- Avoid prolonged standing with straight legs. During prolonged standing, one foot should be kept over a low stool and alternated between feet.
- Use of topical OTC creams: Ketoprofen, Ibuprofen, Diclofenac, Lidocaine etc.

Food and back pain: Page:

When to seek medical advice: Page:

Pain due to body stiffness

Muscles feels tight and difficult to move. Movement causes muscle pain. It may involve a small area of the body or a whole body. Stiffness and pain may be mild or severe. Almost all muscle stiffness and pain go away on their own. Sometimes stiffness and pain can stay for longer period.

Causes:

- Muscle sprain and strain of muscle.
- Lifting heavy weights.
- Hard physical work. After exercise.
- Influenza and other viral illness.
- Rheumatoid arthritis.
- Some medications: statin drugs.
- Thyroid gland underactivity.

Home remedies and prevention:

- Taking rest from normal activites for only few days.
- Elevation of the part if possible.
- Cold compression for sudden pain.
- Warm bath for prolonged pain.
- Massage therapy for sore areas
- Maintaining proper hydration of body.
- OTC pain relievers.
- Regular muscle stretching and exercises.
- Always healthy posture is maintained.
- Taking break from work.
- Healthy and balanced diet.

When to seek medical advice:

- Stiffness and pain accompanied by fever.
- Extreme muscle weakness.
- Home remedies donot relieve stiffness and pain.

Knee pain

Knee pain is a common problem among the older adults over the age of 65. The most common cause is osteoarthritis of the knee joint, which is thought to be caused by wear and tear in the joint.

Features of *knee* pain:

- The gap between the two knees gradually increases. The leg looks like a 'bow', with a curve outward to the side.
- Gradual increase of pain, especially during and after walking.
- Knee becomes stiff and range of movements decreases.
- Swelling of the knee and warm to touch.
- Feeling of weakness and instability in the knee.
- Popping / crunching noises heard on movement of the knee.
- Inability to fully straighten and bend the knee.

BODY PAIN AND PAIN RELIEF

Home remedies:

If knee pain is mild to moderate in nature, the following measures may be helpful.

- Remain active with physical activities like walking, swimming in warm pool, cycling, warm pool exercises, etc.
- Muscle strengthening exercises:
    o Leg raising while lying or sitting down.
    o Standing on one foot.
    o Sitting on a chair and then standing repeatedly for a minute. Wall squatting.
- Use of walking aid and/or knee brace.
- Body weight management.
- OTC pain relievers: Ibuprofen, Naproxen, Ketoprofen.
- Keeping a healthy and balanced diet.
- Massage of the muscles and tissues around the knees. Massage should be done in a seated position with the knee pointing forward and the feet flat on the floor.
- Heat therapy in the knees. Benefits: page.

Prevention of knee pain:

- Maintenance of a healthy body weight.
- Stretching of the muscles around the knee.
- Exercises to increase strength of muscles around the knees.
- Continuing to perform personal activities of daily living.
- Knees should be kept flexible by maintaining an active life.
- Walking aid may be used.
- A healthy and balanced diet.
- Completing activities in a warm pool. Benefits: page.

When to seek medical advice:

- Severe pain in the knee and inability to fully bend or straighten the knee, and/or inability to bear weight on the knee.
- Feeling of the knee 'giving out' while walking.
- An obvious deformity of the knee.
- Knee pain associated with fever.

also see knee pain: page.

Neck pain

Neck pain is common among older adults. The most common cause of neck pain in older adults is inflammation of the joints in the neck, called cervical spondylosis or inflammation of shoulder joints. Due to the inflammation, the cervical nerves become pinched between the bones. Osteoarthritis of neck joints is another major cause of neck pain.

Features of neck pain. See neck pain page.

Home remedies and prevention. See neck pain page.

When to seek medical advice: See neck pain page.

Muscle pain: Polymyalgia rheumatica

Muscular pain due to polymyalgia rheumatica (PMR) is common among older adults. PMR occurs due to inflammation of tissues around joints, causing pain and stiffness in the joints. *Shoulders* and *hips* are typically most affected, but PMR may occur across the entire body. The pain may start as an acute attack or can occur gradually over a longer period. Most people with PMR wake-up in the morning with pain in their muscles, that become better as the day progresses. However, sometimes the pain and stiffness persists all day long.

Causes of PMR: See page 302.

Features of PMR: See page 302.

Home remedies and prevention of PMR: See page 304.

When to seek medical advice: See page 304.

Muscle pain: Fibromyalgia

Fibromyalgia is characterized by widespread musculoskeletal pain and stiffness across multiple body sites accompanied by fatigue. Fibromyalgia can occur at any age and in both women and men. Typically fibromyalgia is triggered by an acute stressful event like physical stress or emotional stress. Fibromyalgia reduces overall quality of life.

Features: See page 161.

BODY PAIN AND PAIN RELIEF

Prevention and home remedies: See page 161.

Complications of fibromyalgia: See page 161.

When to seek medical advice: See page 161.

Hip pain

Hip pain is a common complaint among older adults. Sometimes, hip pain is accompanied by back pain and other joint pain.

Most common causes of hip pain.

- *Osteoarthritis:* see page:
- *Rheumatoid arthritis:* See page:
- *Tendonitis:* Inflammation of tendons around the hip joint.
- *Bursitis:* Inflammation of bursa around the hip joint.
- *Strain* and *sprain* of muscles and tendons around the hip.
- *Septic arthritis:* Infection of the hip joint. See page:
- *Tumors* of the bone and/or soft tissue around the hip joint.
- *Necrosis* of bone due to reduced blood supply.

Features of hip pain: See hip pain: page 229.

Home remedies and prevention of hip pain:

There is no magic cure for pain and stiffness of osteoarthritis of the hip. However, there are a number of ways to reduce the pain and stiffness and return to a reasonably normal lifestyle.

- Remain physically active. Rest is not the only answer.
- Continue activities of daily life.
- Low impact exercise is advised such as walking, cycling, and warm pool swimming.
- Maintaining of a healthy body weight.
- A healthy and balanced diet is beneficial: chart
- Use of walking aids:
    o Hand stick. Crutches. Braces.
    o Soft walking shoes. Shoe inserts if necessary. OTC pain relievers: Ibuprofen, Naproxen, Acetaminophen.
- OTC topical analgesics may be used.

- Applying heat compression to the joints.
- Stretching and strengthening exercises for the hip and thigh muscles.

When to seek medical advice for hip pain: See page 228.

Osteoporosis and body pain in old age: See page

Headache in older adults

Like other sources of body pain, headaches are also a distressing symptom among older adults. The most common causes of headache are tension headache and migraine. Intracranial lesions may also cause headache in older adults.

Tension headaches

Tension headaches are the most common type of headache among the adults and teens. They cause mild to moderate pain and come and go over time, typically with no other symptoms.

Features of:

tension headache: page

Migraine headaches. page

Headache due to brain tumour. page

Home remedies for common headaches:

- Adequate hydration by drinking water, sports drinks etc.
- Adequate sleep. Cold compress.
- Healthy and balanced diet. chart.
- Avoid food with high histamine: chart.
- Food supplementation with calcium, Vitamin D, Magnesium, Vitamin B-complex etc.

See also page: 224.

Hand and finger pain in older adults

Hand and finger pain is a common complaint among older adults. The majority of causes are age related degeneration and inflammation. Unfortunately, age related degenerative changes in the musculoskeletal, vascular, and nervous system are inevitable. These changes are accompanied by:

- Osteoarthritis page
- Rheumatoid arthritis page
- Osteoporosis. page
- Tendonitis (inflammation in the tissuses which connect muscles to the bones).
- Inflammation of bursa (bursitis). Bursas are fluid filled sacs around joints which act as a cushion for ligaments' and tendons' movements.
- Nerve compression symptoms.

Features of hand and finger pain:

- Dull or burning pain in small joints of hands and fingers.
- Pain at rest or with movements of joints.
- Joint stiffness. Stiffness may be marked in the morning or after a period of inactivity.
- Swelling around joints.
- Sensation of grinding, grating or looseness around finger joints.
- Tingling and numbness in hands.
- Decreased grip strength.
- Joint deformity.

Home remedies for hand and finger pain:

Unfortunately, there is no cure for inflammatory arthritis in the hand. The following may help to keep pain from impeding on day-to-day activities:

- Splinting of the hand and wrist by a brace to give rest to the hand during an acute pain attack.
- Heat therapy, movements of fingers in warm water.
- Moderate exercises for the fingers. The fingers should be kept mobile and range of movement exercise for fingers is adviced. Exercises can help to keep the supportive ligaments and tendons in hands flexible and may help to reduce pain in hands.
- OTC pain relievers: Ibuprofen, Naproxen, Ketoprofen.

Prevention of hand and finger pain:

Majority cases of arthritis are not preventable and cannot be cured, but the appearance of symptoms can be delayed.

- Patient must stay active.
- Activities of daily living should be continued.
- Prolonged rest is not beneficial.
- Regular exercises of the hand will reduce pain and stiffness, especially if the person already has arthritis.
- Taking of regular advice from physician will help to delay symptoms.

See also hand pain, page 169 and finger pain, page 201.

Foot and ankle pain in older adults

The feet support the weight of the body and undergo a lot of wear and tear. As we age, most of the body tissues tend to shrink, while the feet seem to grow larger. This is due to years of standing, walking, and exercising. With time, the arches fall, the joints stiffen and the padding on the bottom of the foot thins. In older age groups, foot problems can become a more frequent occurrence.

The most common foot problems in older adults include:

- Bunions. see foot and heel pain: page
- Corns. foot and heel pain: page
- Calluses. foot and heel pain: page
- Hammer toes.
- Ingrown toe nails. foot and heel pain. page
- Diabetic foot. see page
- Inflammation of soft tissues on the sole of the foot.
- Foot ischemia: reduced blood to the foot.
- Inflammation of Achilles' tendon. The Achilles' tendon is a tough band of tissue that connects the calf muscles to the heel bone.

Factors aggravating foot and heel pain:

- Uncontrolled diabetes mellitus.
- Walking barefooted on hard surfaces.
- Hard and ill-fitted shoes and slippers.
- Abnormal shape of the foot and heel.

BODY PAIN AND PAIN RELIEF

- Excess bodyweight.
- Unhealthy foot hygiene.

Plantar fascia:

Features of inflammation of the *plantar fascia*.page: foot and heel pain

Features of inflammation of *Achilles' tendon*. see page foot and heel pain

Features of inflammation of foot joints:

- *Pain* in the ankle and foot during walking and at rest.
- *Swelling* around the joint.
- *Stiffness* of the ankle and foot.
- *Deformity* of ankle joint. Lumpy ankle joint.
- *Tingling* and *numbness* in the foot and toes.

Prevention of foot pain:

- Use of well-fitted, well-cushioned, and comfortable footwear.
- High heel and narrow toed shoes should be avoided.
- Healthy and good foot hygiene practice.
- Never to walk barefooted.
- Healthy body weight should be maintained.
- Diabetes should be strictly controlled.
- Stretching should be done before exercise.

Maintenance of good foot hygiene:

- Feet should be kept as clean as the face.
- Use of gentle soap to clean the feet.
- Make sure to clean between the toes.
- Feet must be dried well before putting on socks. Moisture-wicking socks are better. Socks should be clean and dry. Anti-fungal powder may be used prior to donning socks.
- Moisturizer may be applied before going to bed.
- Nails should be trimmed regularly but must not cut them too short and must not be cut-back to prevent ingrown toenails.

When to seek medical advice:

- Pain following a trauma to the foot.
- Pain is not relieved by at-home therapies.

- Pain that is accompanied by fever, redness and swelling.
- Unable to perform normal walking patterns.
- Pain persists for more than a week.
- Sleep disturbances due to pain.
- Severe pain and swelling in the foot.

See also foot and heel pain page: 209.

Bone Infection and Pain

Bone infection, or osteomyelitis, is a painful condition common in children, but can occur at any age. Any bone in the body may be affected. Generally, the infecting germs travel through the blood stream from a distant site in the body to the bone and establish an infection. The infection destroys the bone and produces symptoms, including pain. Organisms may also reach the bone by a direct injury to the bone, causing the bone exposed to the exterior and to germs.

Risk factors for bone *infection:*

- Trauma to the bone.
- Long term skin and oral infections:
    - Boils, furuncles, carbuncles, etc.
    - Dental infections.
- Uncontrolled or poorly controlled diabetes.
- Poor blood circulation due to:
    - High blood pressure. Diabetes of long duration.
    - High blood cholesterol causing narrowing of blood vessels.
- Heavy smoking.
- Immunosuppressive drugs use and abuse.
- Chronic kidney failure and hemodialysis.
- Severe anemia.
- Intravenous therapy.
- Intravenous drug use and abuse.

Common sites of bone *infection:*

- Growing areas of bone in children.
- Bones in the spine in adult.
- Hip bones.
- Small bones of feet.
- Long bones of arms and legs.

BODY PAIN AND PAIN RELIEF

Features of bone infection:

- Pain and swelling in the area of the bone infection.
- Redness of skin over the swelling and warm to touch.
- Irritability or general feeling of being unwell.
- Fever and chills. Feeling of lethargy and weakness.
- Stiffness or inability to use the affected limb.
- Drainage of pus or foul smelling fluid from the affected area.

When to seek medical advice:

As soon as a bone infection is suspected, it is best to consult an orthopedic surgeon.

Bone Tumor and Body Pain

Bone is composed of proteins, primarily collagen, and minerals, primarily calcium as well as phosphorus, magnesium, sodium and bicarbonate. Together these materials give bone a unique combination of strength and elasticity. A bone tumor is an abnormal growth of tissue in bone and develop when cells within a bone multiply in an uncontrollable manner. Tumors form a lump or mass of abnormal tissue. As the tumor grows, abnormal tissue displace the healthy tissue. Tumors can be benign (not cancerous) or malignant (cancerous).

Benign (non-cancerous) bone tumors

Most bone tumors are benign, are not cancerous. They are usually not life-threatening. They typically stay in the same place where they start and do not spread to other bones or other parts of the body. Though benign tumors grow slowly, they require treatment. Benign tumors can grow to a large mass of tissue, compressing the surrounding healthy tissue and causing symptoms. Benign bone tumors are mostly observed in children when their skeleton is still growing.

Malignant (cancerous) bone tumors

Malignant tumors are cancerous and rare. These tumors are generally rapid growing and cause local tissue destruction. They can spread to distant organs throughout the body.

Causes of bone tumor:

- Exact cause is unknown.
- There are genetic factors that can pass within families.
- Radiation therapy and use of anti-cancer drugs.

Features of *benign* bone tumors:

- A lump or swelling over a bone, which is growing very slowly. Increasing pain in the region of the tumor.
- Fracture of the bone and features of bone fracture.

BODY PAIN AND PAIN RELIEF

Features of *malignant* bone tumors:

- Bone pain that becomes worse at night.
- Pain that is not relieved by OTC pain relievers.
- Rapidly increasing swelling or a lump in the affected area.
- Pain to touch over the affected area.
- Gradual loss of appetite.
- Unintended weight loss.
- Generalized weakness and fatigue.
- Bone gradually weakens and ultimately fracture occurs in the affected area.

When to seek medical advice:

As soon as a bone tumor is suspected, it is best to consult an orthopedic surgeon.

Chest Pain

'Only do what your heart tells you'

- Princess Diana

Chest pain is a pain or discomfort in the chest, typically in the front part of the chest wall. It may be described as sharp stab, dull ache, pressure, heaviness or squeezing, crushing or burning. Associated symptoms include pain in the shoulder, arm, upper abdomen, neck or jaw. Pain may be associated with nausea, sweating, or shortness of breath. Chest pain may or may not be heart related. The majority of chest pain (70%) is non-heart related, with the remaining 30% being heart related.

In adults, the most common causes of chest pain include:

Non-heart related causes (70%)

- Gastrointestinal (stomach, intestines) 40%.
  - Food pipe (esophagus), heartburn, acid reflux from stomach.
  - Stomach ulcer.
  - Pancreas, inflammation of the pancreas.
- Musculoskeletal (muscles, bones, joints) 30%.
  - Muscle strain from exertion.
  - Diseases of the spine, including cervical angina.
  - Injured or broken ribs (chest wall bones).
  - Costochondritis: inflammation of cartilage of ribs.
  - Nerve compression.
- Lung-related 1-2%.
  - Bronchitis: infection and inflammation of airway tube.
  - Pneumonia: inflammation of the lungs.
  - Pleuritis: inflammation of the covering of lung and inner chest wall.
  - Pneumothorax: air between the chest wall and lungs.

- o Pulmonary embolism: blockage of pulmonary artery by blood clot or air.
- o Bronchospasm: constriction of air passages in asthma.

Heart-related causes (30%)

- *Coronary artery disease.*
  - o Angina occurs due to narrowed (rather than blocked) coronary arteries of heart.
  - o Heart attack: blood flow to the heart is blocked (coronary artery completely blocked).
- Other heart related causes: 1-2%.
  - o *Pericarditis:* inflammation of the sac around the heart.
  - o *Myocarditis:* inflammation of the heart muscle.
  - o *Cardiomyopathy:* a disease of the heart muscle.
  - o Aortic dissection: a tear in the aorta (large artery).

Chest pain in children

- Musculoskeletal 70%.
- Exercise induced 10%.
- Gastrointestinal 10%.
- Psychogenic 5%.
- Others 5%.

Non-heart related or non-cardiac chest pain

Non-cardiac chest pain is the term that is used to describe pain in the chest that is not caused by heart diseases or a heart attack. In most people (70%), non-cardiac chest pain is related to the following organs:

- *Esophagus:* the tube that connects the mouth with the stomach.
- *Muscles or bones* in the chest, chest wall or spine (back).
- *Lung diseases.*
- *Stomach* problems, such as stomach ulcers or tumors.
- *Pancreas* problems, such as inflammation of the pancreas.
- Stress.
- Anxiety and depression.

Features of *non-cardiac* chest pain:

- Chest pain often described as the same feeling as the chest pain caused by heart disease.
- Heartburn creates a burning sensation behind the breast bone (sternum).
- Symptoms of acid reflux disease can occur at the same time as heartburn. These can include nausea, bloating, and belching.
- A sour taste or a sensation of food re-entering the mouth.
- Pain on swallowing or eating.
- Trouble in swallowing.
- Pain that gets better or worse when body position is changed.
- Pain that intensifies when breathing deeply or coughing.
- Tenderness when chest is pushed.
- Fever and chills.
- Pain that persists for many hours.
- Panic or anxiety.

Pain related to the esophagus

The esophagus connects the mouth to the stomach. The contents of the stomach are acidic, which is corrosive in nature and can cause tissue injury. When the contents of the stomach move back up into the esophagus and throat, it can cause a burning feeling in the chest and a sour taste in the mouth. After intense vomiting, an esophageal tear may occur and result in sudden and intense chest pain.

Heart burn

Heart burn is a symptom, not a disease. It is the sensation, usually of burning pain, caused by acid reflux. Acid reflux occurs when the acidic contents of the stomach splashes back up into the esophagus. Heartburn is not related to the heart in any way. The confusion comes from the location of the pain in the chest.

The stomach produces mucus to protect its lining from the acid that it uses to help with digestion, however the esophagus lacks the proper mucus protection. Due to this lack of protection, acid reflux can damage lining of the esophagus and causes pain behind the breastbone (sternum). This pain is due to acid-sensitive nerves present in the esophagus.

Features of heartburn:

- Heartburn creates a burning sensation behind the breastbone (sternum).
- The burning-type pain typically occurs in the upper central region of abdomen (epigastric region). The acid can also reach higher up, possibly even as far as the back of the mouth.
- Other symptoms of acid reflux disease can appear with the heartburn including nausea, bloating and belching.

Differences between features of *heartburn* and *heart attack*.

It can sometimes be difficult to know if symptoms are due to a heart attack or heartburn.

The main differences between the symptoms are:

- Heartburn tends to be worse after eating and when lying down, but a heart attack can happen without a relation to eating. Lying down aggravates the pain in heart attack, while sitting up and leaning forwards often relieves the pain.
- Heartburn can be relieved by drugs that reduce acid levels in the stomach, such as antacids etc.
- Heartburn usually does not cause other general symptoms, such as breathlessness.
- Heart attack does not cause bloating or belching, but these can happen with heartburn.

Pain related to stomach ulcers

The stomach is an abdominal organ. Stomach ulcers are sores in the stomach lining. Stomach ulcer pain is burning or gnawing pain in the upper central region of abdomen, known as the epigastric region. They usually do not cause intense pain. However, they can cause a recurring discomfort in the chest. Taking antacids, which are OTC drugs, can usually relieve pain.

Stomach ulcers in detail: see page 12.

Pain related to the muscles in the chest wall

This type of pain is caused by muscle strain and inflammation of tendons around the ribs, causing persistent chest pain. If the pain becomes worse with activity, then it may be a symptom of a muscle strain. Fibromyalgia can produce persistent muscle-related chest pain.

Common features of *chest wall muscle pains*:

- Sharp aching and stabbing pain in the chest.
- Pain on breathing.
- Pain becomes worse upon movement of the chest and twisting the trunk.
- Raising the arms increases pain.
- Deep breathing, sneezing, and coughing increases pain.
- There may be a history of trauma to the chest wall.

Home remedies for chest wall muscle pain:

- Complete rest. As soon as pain is noticed all activities should be stopped.
- Strenuous exercises, like heavy lifting should be avoided.
- Application of cold pack to the affected area is soothing.
- Massage to the chest wall.
- Analgesic cream (an OTC drug) may be used.
- Assuming a half lying position is the best. In this position, the body is bent at the hips and the trunk is raised from lying position to any angle between 45° to 90°. Sleeping in a recliner may help.
- OTC pain relievers: Ibuprofen, Acetaminophen, Naproxen.

When to seek medical advice:

It is important to seek medical advice to exclude heart and lung related pain. Therefore it is important to seek medical advice when pain in the chest is accompanied by:

- Sweating. Rapid pulse.
- Difficulty in breathing.
- Lightheadedness. Dizziness. Nausea.
- Irritability. Fainting.
- Fever.
- Sleepiness.

Pain related to injured ribs

Injuries to the ribs, such as bruises, breaks and fractures can cause chest pain. This typically occurs due to a history of trauma to the chest wall and the pain tends to be extreme.

As soon as injury to the ribs is suspected, the patient must seek medical advice.

Pain related to costochondritis

Costochondritis, an inflammation of the cartilage of chest cage, can cause chest pain. The pain is sharp, aching or pressure-like. There is tenderness in the chest wall, that is, the chest is painful to the touch or pressure and this finding is diagnostic for this condition. This type of pain may get worse when sitting or lying in certain positions. Pain also occurs when a person does any physical activity.

Home remedies for costochondritis:

- Complete bed rest in a reclining position.
- Application of a heating pad to the painful area.
- OTC pain relievers: ibuprofen, naproxen, acetaminophen.
- Analgesic cream application.

When to seek medical advice:

Medical advice should be sought to rule out heart and lung-related pains and infection in the area.

Following features indicate that the medical advice is urgent.

- Intense chest pain.
- Difficulty in breathing.
- Lightheadedness. Dizziness.
- Fever. Sweating. Rapid pulse.
- Nausea and vomitting.
- Irretability. Fainting.

Pain related to lung diseases.

Pneumonia

Pneumonia is an infection and inflammation of the lung tissues. The infection occurs in the air sacs or alveoli, and due to the infection, the air sacs are filled with fluid or purulent material and produces symptoms. Pneumonia may be life threatening.

Features of pneumonia:

- Chest pain on breathing and coughing.
- Pain may be sharp or stabbing in character.
- Coughing out of greenish, yellow or bloody mucus.
- Shortness of breath.
- Fever, sweating and chills.
- Fever may be absent in old and debilitated patients.
- Feeling of fatigue and very tired.
- Headache.
- Changes in mental awareness in older patients.

When to seek medical advice:

If pneumonia is suspected, immediate medical advice is a mandatory.

Home remedies for some of the symptoms of pneumonia:

First, patients must seek medical advice for pneumonia. Here home remedies are given for some mild symptoms of pneumonia.

- Sufficient physical and mental rest.
- Healthy and balanced diet.
- Drinking lots of warm water and warm tea.
- If shortness of breath is present:
    o Steam inhalation.
    o Warm black or green tea.
    o One or two cups of coffee.
    o Warm and dump air for breathing is beneficial.
- Saline water gargle for cough.
- Chest pain due to repeated cough:
    o Warm ginger and turmeric tea.

- o OTC pain relievers: Acetaminophen.Naproxen.
- Fever:
  - o Proper hydration.
  - o OTC fever and pain relievers.
  - o A lukewarm bath or compress.
- Chills:Drinking of warm plain water, herbal teas, soup.
- To boost immune system:
  - o Garlic. Raw honey. Green tea.
  - o Cayenne pepper. Echinacea.

Pulmonary embolism

Pulmonary arteries carry blood from the heart to the lungs. One pulmonary trunk,which is a large tube and arises from the heart. Pulmonary trunk divides into two pulmonary arteries and carries blood to both lungs. In pulmonary embolism, the pulmonary artery or its branches are blocked. Generally, this blockage is caused by blood clots that travel to the heart from deep veins situated in the legs or other parts of the body. From the heart, the clots travel to the lungs and block blood supply to the lungs. This blockage is called a pulmonary embolism and is a life threatening condition.

Features of pulmonary embolism:

- Sudden shortness of breath that gets worse with physical activity and exertion.
- Sharp pain in the chest like a heart attack pain.
- Deep breathing increases the intensity of pain.
- Pain becomes worse on coughing, bending forwards, or stooping.
- Difficulty in breathing.
- Coughing of blood-streaked sputum.
- Rapid and irregular heart rate.
- Excessive sweating. Clammy skin.
- Fever.
- Patient may have leg pain caused by deep vein thrombosis.

Prevention of pulmonary embolism:

- Maintenance of a healthy body weight.
- Avoidance of prolonged rest in bed or chair.
- Use of compression stockings in the legs.
- Stretching of leg and foot during long flights.

- At least one minute of walking in every hour of sitting or lying is beneficial.
- Avoidence of smoking.
- Strictly control of diabetes and hypertension.

When to seek medical advice:

Pulmonary embolism is a life threatening condition. Urgent medical treatment is mandatory to save life and to exclude heart related pain.

It is important to be careful and to consult a physician for any of the following situations as they can be related to pulmonary embolisms more frequently:

- Obese and overweight patients.
- Oral contraceptives user.
- Hormone replacement therapy (HRT) receiver.
- long-term smoker.
- Diabetes, controlled or uncontrolled.
- High blood pressure.
- Long term kidney disease.
- Heart failure.
- Family history of pulmonary embolism.
- Cancer anywhere in the body.
- Chemotherapy receiver patients.
- Pregnancy.

Pain related to lung airways

A common airway disease is *bronchial asthma*. Bronchial asthma is a chronic inflammatory disease of the airways which causes the airway path of the lungs to swell and narrow. Inflammation also causes the pathway to produce excess mucus, making it narrower and hard to breathe. Bronchial asthma results in periodic 'attacks' of coughing, wheezing, shortness of breath and chest tightness. Bronchial asthma is a chronic disease and interferes with the activities of daily life.

Features of bronchial asthma:

- Difficulty in breathing, especially when exhaling.
- Chest tightness.
- Chest pain. Shortness of breath.
- Coughing, especially during exertion.

- Wheezing: a whistling or squeaky sound in the chest when breathing, especially when exhaling.

Common risk factors and triggers of an asthma attack:

- Family history of asthma.
- Bad air quality, precense of dust, pollen, dust mites.
- Respiratory infections.
- Smoking. Certain fragrances and foods.
- Strenuous physical activity or exercise.
- Changes in weather, cold or chilly air.
- Exposure to harmful chemical fumes.
- Medications including beta-blockers, NSAIDS.
- Pet dander: microscopic flecks of skin shed by dogs, cats, birds and other animals.
- Cockroach droppings and fragments.
- Being overweight or obese.
- Food preservatives. Food allergy.

Home remedies and prevention of asthma attacks:

- Identification and avoidance of asthma triggers and allergens.
- Foods which cause symptoms should be marked, noted, and avoided.
- Avoiding smoke of any type.
- Avoiding steam baths.
- Taking of preventive measures against weather changes.
    - Exercise should be done safely with asthma.
    - Good exercise includes:
        - Low-impact walking. Biking. Swimming in warm pool. Golf. Baseball. Racquet sports.
- Get vaccinated against allergens and viruses.
- Immunotherapy.
- Yoga and mindfulness.
- Asthma medications are taken as per physician advice.
- Maintaining contact with healthcare workers.

Several types of foods are common allergens. Any foods that cause allergic reactions should be avoided.

Common foods *allergens:*

- o Shrimp and other shellfish. Eggs.
- o Preserved foods. Peanuts.
- o Cow's milk.
- o Salty foods. Mixed salads.
- o Soy foods. Wheat.
  - Foods *beneficial* in asthma:
  - Fresh fruits and vegetables.
  - Vitamin D rich foods: chart.
  - Vitamin C rich foods: chart.
  - Vitamin E supplements.
  - Omega-3 fatty acid rich foods. chart.
  - Beta-carotene rich vegetables: chart.
  - Magnesium-rich foods: chart.
  - Tea. Coffee. Avocado. Milk and egg, if not allergic
  - Honey, Garlic, Ginger and Turmeric.

Emergency asthma treatment at home:

It is safe to seek medical advice as soon as possible. Until medical help can be sought, the following guidance may be used:

- Remain calm and quiet.
- Stand or sit up straight. Do not lie down.
- If preferred to be in bed, remain in a propped-up position.
- One or two puffs may be taken.
- Sipping warm black tea or coffee is beneficial.
- Inhale steam.
- Pursed lip breathing: Breathe-in through the nose and out through the pursed lips. Exhale should be longer than the inhale.
- Seek medical help as soon as possible.

When to seek medical advice:

- Pain in the chest and difficulty in breathing.
- Severe breathlessness or wheezing, especially at night or in the morning.
- Feeling of tightness in the chest.
- Inability to speak more than short phrases due to shortness of breath. Rapid breathing.
- Having to strain chest muscles to breathe.

- Blue lips and fingernails.
- Feeling confused, agitated, or exhausted.
- Getting no relief from using reliever inhaler.
- Very rapid breathing, coughing, wheezing or gasping.
- Fainting or collapsing.

Pain related to covering of lungs. Inflammation of pleura (pleurisy)

The covering of the lung is called the *pleura*. Pleura has two layers. One layer of the pleura covers the lungs and the other layer covers the inner chest wall. Between these two layers is a potential space, called the pleural space, which is usually filled with very small amount of liquid. This liquid helps the two layers to glide between them during breathing.

Inflammation of the pleura (pleurisy) will cause pain due to the friction between the pleural layers. Pleural pain is marked during inhalation and exhalation, and the pain lessens or stops when breath is held willingly.

Features of pleurisy:

- Typically pain is on one side of the chest.
- Pain is sharp when breathing is deep, while coughing or while sneezing.
- Pain may be felt in shoulders and back.
- Shallow breathing is used to avoid feeling of pain.
- Pain is relieved by taking shallow breaths.
- Shortness of breath.
- Dry cough.
- Muscles and joints pain.
- Headache.

When to seek medical advice:

It is safest to seek medical advice as soon as pleurisy is suspected.

Pain related to collapsed lung
When air builds up in the space between the lung and the chest wall, the lung collapses.

Features of a collapsed lung:

- Sudden chest pain when breathing.
- Shortness of breath.
- Rapid breathing. Rapid heart rate.
- Feeling of fatigueness.

When to seek medical advice:

As soon as a collapsed lung is suspected, it is best to seek medical advice.

Pain related to high blood pressure in the lung (pulmonary hypertension)
High blood pressure in the arteries that carry blood to the lung tissue is called pulmonary hypertension.

Features of pulmonary hypertension:

- Shortness of breath.
- Chest pain. Heart palpitations: rapid heart rate.
- Fatigue. Feeling faint.
- Swelling in the legs, ankles, feet or abdomen.

When to seek medical advice:

As soon as pulmonary hypertention is suspected, medical advice should be sought.

Pain related to the sac around the heart
Sac around the heart is called *pericardium*.

Inflammation of the sac around the heart is called *pericarditis*.

Features of *pericarditis*:

- Sharp or stabbing chest pain. Sometimes pain may be dull, achy, or pressure-like.
- Pain may be felt behind the breast bone (sternum) or in the left side of the chest.
- Pain may spread to the left shoulder and neck.
- Pain often gets worse while coughing, lying down or during a deep breath.
- Sitting up and leaning forward lessens the pain.
- Fever. Cough. Rapid heart rate.
- Shortness of breath while lying down.
- Abdominal or leg swelling.
- General feeling of fatigue.

When to seek medical advice:

As soon as pericarditis is suspected, you *must seek* medical advice.

Pain related to pancreas
The pancreas is an abdominal organ and inflammation of pancreas is called pancreatitis. Pancreatitis may cause pain in the lower chest and pain is made worse by lying down flat.

Pain related to pancreas: see page 35.

Pain related to neck (cervical spine)
Pain in the neck (cervical spine) is called 'cervical angina' and is one potential cause of non-cardiac chest pain. It originates from disorders of the cervical spine.

See neck pain: page 282.

Pain in the chest related to a panic attack
A *panic attack* is an acute anxiety, terror, or fright that is usually of sudden onset. Panic attack typically peaks in 10 minutes or less, and may be uncontrollable.

Panic attack is characterized by:

- Heart palpitations (rapid heart rate).
- Sweating.
- Feeling of shortness of breath and choking.
- Chest pain or discomfort.
- Nausea or abdominal distress.

Home remedies for panic attacks:

- The patient must themselves recognize that it is a panic attack, and not a heart attack. Patient must understand that, the attack is temporary, and it will pass soon.
- Deep breathing exercises, such as breathe deeply through the nose.
- Remaining physically active.
- Gentle and light exercises, such as walking and swimming.
- Closing the eyes for a short period is helpful as it will reduce potential visual stimuli which may causing the panic attack.
- Smoking and alcohol should be avoided.
- Meditation and mindfulness is advised and should be practiced.
- A deep focus on a favorite object will help.
- Muscle relaxation techniques can help to stop panic attacks.
- Turning the mind to a happy place will reduce the feelings of the panic attack.

When to seek medical advice for panic attack:

Panic attacks may become worse without treatment. So, as soon as panic attack is suspected, seek medical care right away.

Heart-related or cardiac chest pain.
Chest pain is often associated with heart diseases, however many people with heart disease present with vague discomfort that is not necessarily identified as pain.

Here, chest discomfort related to a heart attack or another heart problem is discussed.

Coronary arteries (arteries of heart itself).

The coronary arteries are the arterial blood vessels of coronary circulation. There are two main coronary arteries, the right and the left coronary arteries. Coronary arteries arise from the aorta (a large artery) of the heart and transport oxygen enriched blood to the muscles of the heart itself.

Heart veins drain away the de-oxygenated blood from the heart muscles and form a large vein called the coronary sinus, which opens in the right chamber (right atrium) of the heart.

The heart muscles require a steady and continuous supply of oxygen to survive and function. Therefore, any condition which reduces or blocks blood transport to the heart will cause pain in the chest and other symptoms.

Following are the coronary artery diseases.

Angina: angina occurs due to narrowed (rather than blocked) coronary arteries of the heart. Here oxygenated blood supply to the heart is reduced.

Heart attack: heart attack occurs when oxygenated blood flow to the heart in the coronary arteries is blocked.

Angina

Angina means to choke or to prevent respiration by compressing or obstructing the air passage.

Angina occurs due to narrowed (rather than blocked) coronary arteries of heart. Narrowed coronary arteries reduce the quantity of oxygenated blood transported to the heart muscle and is a symptom of coronary artery disease. Although angina is relatively common, it can be hard to distinguish from other types of chest pain, such as the discomfort of indigestion or pain due to chest wall trauma or a muscle pull. Unexplained chest pain must be immediately examined and investigated by a physician to exclude a heart-related chest pain.

Risk factors for angina:

- Family history of heart disease and high blood pressure.
- Diabetes mellitus.
- High blood pressure.
- Smoking. Obesity
- High blood cholesterol.
- Age over 55.
- Sedentary lifestyle and lack of exercise.
- Excess stress and anger.

Features of angina:

- Chest pain and discomfort. The pain is often described as squeezing, burning, pressure, heaviness, tightness or fullness in the chest. It may feel like a vise is squeezing the chest or a heavy weight has been placed on the chest. Pain may radiate to the arms, neck, jaw, shoulder or back.
- Nausa
- Shortness of breath. Cold sweat.
- Dizziness. Fatigue.

Features are need to be evaluated immediately by a physician.

Angina may be sub-divided into:

o Stable angina, and
o Unstable angina.

Stable angina

Stable angina is the most common form of angina and generally occurs due to exertion and goes away with the rest. It is due to hard work of the heart, such as physical exercise, climbing stairs or walking uphill.

Features of *stable angina:*

- Triggers of stable angina include physical activity, emotional stress, cold temperature, heavy meals and smoking. It can be predicted prior to the attack occurring, and the pain is similar to other types of chest pain.
- Lasts for a short time, perhaps five minutes or less.
- Pain disappears with rest or taking angina medications.

Unstable angina

Unstable angina is a medical emergency and can be a precursor to a heart attack. It requires an emergency management.

Features of unstable angina:

- Chest pain is unexpected and can even start at rest.
- It does not follow the typical pattern of angina.
- Unstable angina is more severe and lasts longer than a stable angina, lasting 30 minutes or more.
- May not disappear with rest or use of angina medications.
- Unstable angina may signal a heart attack.

Immediate management of an anginal attack:

- Complete stoppage of all physical activities.
- Mental relaxation and physical rest.
- To *lie down on the floor* or bed, if possible.
- To take a nitroglycerine inhaler.
- If the pain or discomfort doesn't stop after taking nitroglycerine, or if symptoms become more severe, call for immediate medical assistance.

Prevention of anginal attack:

- Smoking and alcohol should be strictly avoided.
- Control of hypertension, diabetes, and high blood cholesterol.
- Healthy and balanced diet. chart.
- Increasing physical activity.
- Reducing stress and anger.
- Maintenance of healthy body weight. chart.

Heart attack / Heart muscle necrosis or death (Myocardial infarction)

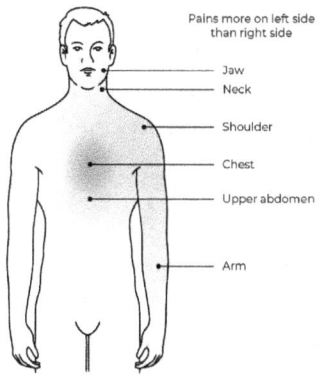

Pain associated with heart attack

A heart attack occurs when the flow of oxygenated blood to the heart is blocked. Decreased oxygen supply to the heart muscle will cause heart muscle death. This condition may be associated with one or more of the following features:

- Chest pain or discomfort of varying degrees.
- Pressure, heaviness, fullness, burning, squeezing sensations, tightness, or ache in the chest.
- Chest pain that feels like a very heavy weight is crushing against the chest.
- Crushing or searing pain that radiates to the back, neck, jaw, shoulders and/or one or both arms.
- The chest pain or discomfort is usually central or slightly to the left of the centre. The pain may also spread to other areas.
- Pain that lasts for more than a few minutes, gets worse with activities, goes away and returns, or varies in intensity.
- Light-headedness, weakness, or fainting.
- Shortness of breath.
- Excessive sweating, including the feeling of 'cold sweats'.
- Dizziness.
- Sudden fatigue, nausea or vomiting, and weakness.

Not all heart attacks give the same symptoms. Symptoms can be mild or severe, while others may experience no symptoms at all.

Distinguishing heart attack pain from other types of chest pain.

Sometimes it can be difficult to distinguish heart-related chest pain from other types of chest pain. However, chest pain that is less likely due to a problem with the heart (non-heart related pain) is more often associated with the following features:

- A sour taste or a sensation of food re-entering the mouth.
- Trouble in swallowing and/or pain with swallowing or eating. Pain that changes when body position is changed.
- Pain that intensifies when breathing deeply or coughing.
- Feeling of pain when chest wall is pushed (tenderness in the chest wall).
- Fever and chills.
- Pain that is persistently present for many hours.
- Panic or anxiety.

The classic symptoms of heartburn which are a painful and/or burning sensation behind the breastbone (sternum) can be caused by problems with the heart or the stomach as well.

Myocarditis

Infection and inflammation of heart muscle is called myocarditis. Myocarditis has symptoms that are similar to a heart attack.

Common features of myocarditis:

- Chest pain.
- Fever. Rapid heart beat.
- Difficulty in breathing.
- Feeling of fatigue.

Prevention of a heart attack:

- Smoking should be stopped.
- Blood pressure, cholesterol level and diabetes controlled.
- Stress management.
- Regular medical check-ups.

- Maintaining a healthy body weight.
- Regular physical exercises.
- Heart-healthy and balanced diet. See chart.

When to seek medical advice for a heart attack:

- Chest pain or discomfort, such as pressure, squeezing, pain, or fullness that lasts more than a few minutes or that goes away and then returns.
- Pain or discomfort in other parts of the body, e.g, one or both arms, back, jaw, neck or stomach.
- Shortness of breath or 'air hunger' (feeling that there is less air to breathe), prior to or with chest discomfort.
- Cold sweat.
- Nausea and dizziness.
- Feeling unusually tired.

Home remedies for chest pain:

When there is a sharp, intense, and burning sensation in the chest, the first thought that can come to mind is that it is a heart attack, and the person may begin to panic. Though cardiac pain is a probability, especially when pain is felt in the left side, it may not always be the sole reason. There are many causes and the majority are less serious causes. Chest pain does not just hurt. It can also interfere with activities of daily life.

Home remedies for chest pains which are due to non-heart related causes:

Stomach causes

- Drinking of warm/cold plain water.
- Antacids. Ginger.
- Physical exercise.
- Possible triggers should be identified and avoided.

Bone, muscle and joint causes

- Heat/ice therapy.
- OTC pain relievers: Ibuprofen, Naproxen, Acetaminophen.
- Skeletal muscle relaxants.
- Physical exercises.
- Muscle stretching exercises.

BODY PAIN AND PAIN RELIEF

Lung causes
- OTC pain relievers: Ibuprofen, Naproxen, Acetaminophen.
- Changes to body position.
- Breathing more slowly.
- Cough suppressants.
- Breathing exercises.

It may not be very easy to tell the difference between a serious heart-related condition and a benign non-heart related pain. When in doubt, you should always seek medical attention.

A person must receive an *urgent medical care* when he experiences the following features:

- Chest pain which feels crushing, squeezing, or heavy.
- A person suspects that he is having a heart-attack.
- Shortness of breath or 'air-hunger' (feeling that there is less air in the area) is experienced along with chest pain.

There are several things a person can try at home to help alleviate chest pain when it occurs and to prevent future occurences.

The home remedies below should only be used when a person has been examined by a physician and is certain that the chest pain is not caused by something serious, such as a heart attack. These remedies are also not meant for a person with acute anginal pain. **People with acute angina should follow the treatment provided by their physician.**

Garlic
Chewing one or two garlic cloves every morning. Garlic prevents cardiovascular disease and improves blood flow to the heart and relieves chest pain.

Almonds
Almonds may help to prevent heart disease and chest pain. Almonds are rich sources of poly-unsaturated fatty acids which promote cardiac health and also help to reduce cholesterol levels.

Aloe vera juice
Aloe vera can help to strengthen the cardiovascular system, regulate blood cholesterol, lower triglyceride levels, and reduce blood pressure. All of these help in relieving chest pain.

Applying a cold pack
When chest pain is due to a muscle strain from exercise or other activities, or blunt trauma, icing the area with cold pack is a widely accepted method to help to reduce swelling and stop the pain.

Hot drinks
A hot drink may help to eliminate gas and relieve chest pain when it is due to gas or bloating. Hibiscus tea lowers blood pressure and cholesterol.

Apple cider vinegar
Apple cider vinegar prevents acid reflux from the stomach and it is a blood thinner.

Aspirin
Aspirin therapy reduces the clumping action of platelets and prevents clot formation. Clots can block the arteries of the heart muscle. Thus, aspirin helps to prevent the heart attack.

Lying down
When heart pain strikes, lying down immediately with the head elevated above the body may bring some relief. A slightly upright position helps when the pain is due to reflux of acid from the stomach.

Turmeric
Turmeric is rich in curcumin and has anti-inflammatory properties. Turmeric thus helps to reduce inflammation and pain symptoms in the chest. It can also reduce cholesterol, clot formation, and artery plaque build-up and thus prevents heart attack and chest pain.

Ginger
Ginger has anti-inflammatory effects and can reduce chest pain and acid reflux from the stomach.

Vitamins
Vitamin D and vitamin B12 supplementations are beneficial in preventing myocardial infarction or heart attacks.

Basil leaves
Basil contains high levels of vitamin K and magnesium. Magnesium promotes blood flow to the heart and relaxes the blood vessels. Vitamin K prevents the

build-up of cholesterol in the walls of blood vessels. Thus both help in the treatment of cardiac disorders as well as chest pain.

Cayenne pepper

Cayenne pepper contains capsaicin which possesses strong anti-inflammatory properties that help to lessen the intensity of chest pain. It also helps in regulating the blood flow to the heart, thereby preventing heart diseases that may cause chest pain.

Fenugreek seeds

Fenugreek seed has powerful anti-inflammatory and anti-oxident properties that enhance cardiovascular health and prevent chest pain. They promote blood flow to the heart and reduce cholesterol levels.

Other benefits include:

- o Reduces the risk of diabetes.
- o Improves milk production and flow.
- o Accelerates weight loss.
- o Raises testosterone and boost-up sperm count.
- o Regulates blood pressure.

The heart and foods.

Diet plays a major role in heart health and can impact the risk of heart disease. In fact, certain foods can influence blood pressure, triglycerides and cholesterol levels, and inflammation. These all are risk factors for heart disease.

Food-related risk factors include:

- Obesity and physical inactivity.
- High cholesterol level.
- Coronary heart disease.
- High blood pressure.
- Uncontrolled diabetes.

A low saturated fat, high-fiber, high plant-food diet can substantially reduce the risk of developing heart disease.

Heart-healthy foods.

Heart-healthy foods and a well-balanced diet can help to keep heart in good condition and minimize the risk of heart diseases.

Basic principles of heart-healthy foods:

- Processed foods avoided and whole food intake is encouraged.
- A wide variety of fruits and vegetables are included.
- A limited amount of full fat dairy products are advised.
- A limited amount of red and processed meat are advised.
- A limited amount of oily fish are advised each week.
- Healthy fats and oils should be included.
- Nuts, seeds, and legumes should be included.
- Alcohol, added salt, and sugar intake is discouraged.

Examples of *heart-healthy* foods:

- Green leafy and non-starchy vegetables.
- Spinach, kale and other green and colored vegetables which are rich in fibers, vitamins, minerals, and nitrates. These vegetables reduce blood pressure and improve blood vessel functions.
- Whole grains like whole wheat, brown rice, oats, rye, quinoa. These lower cholesterol and systolic blood pressure.
- Fatty fish and fish oils like salmon, mackerel, sardines, and tuna which contain omega-3 fatty acids.
- Beans contain resistant starch and reduce levels of cholesterol and triglycerides, lower blood pressure and act as an anti-inflammatory agent.
- Tomatoes contain lycopene which is a powerful anti-oxidant.
- Walnuts reduces cholesterol and blood pressure.
- Avocados contain mono-unsaturated fats and potassium. They lowers cholesterol, blood pressure and risk of metabolic syndrome.
- Almonds are high in fiber and mono-unsaturated fats, reducing cholesterol and belly fat.
- Seeds, including chia seeds, flaxseeds and hemp seeds contain fiber, and omega-3 fatty acids. Seeds reduce inflammation, blood pressure, cholesterol and triglycerides.
- Dark chocolate contains flavonoids, a powerful anti-oxidant.
- Garlic contains allicin. benefits of garlic, chart.
- Olive oil is rich in anti-oxidant and mono-unsaturated fats. They lowers blood pressure and risk of heart disease.

- Green tea contains polyphenols and catechins. Benefits of green tea, chart.

Functions of anti oxidants: chart.

Functions of omega-3 fatty acids: chart.

Foods bad for the heart.

- Refined carbohydrates and sugar, including white bread, refined rice, and pasta.
- Extra salt in foods and drinks.
- Saturated fat and butter.
- Red meat and processed meat.
- Non-dairy creamer.
- Junk foods such as potato chips, cookies, pies, and ice cream.
- Energy drinks.
- Excess protien.
- Pastries, packaged snacks, fast foods, pizza.

Tips for a healthy heart.

- Maintaining a healthy body weight.
- Eating a healthy and balanced diet.
- Avoiding a full belly.
- Regular physical exercise.
- Avoiding long periods of sitting.
- Smoking cessation.
- Relieving mental stress.

Diabetes and Body Pain

Eating sweet things is not the cause of diabetes.

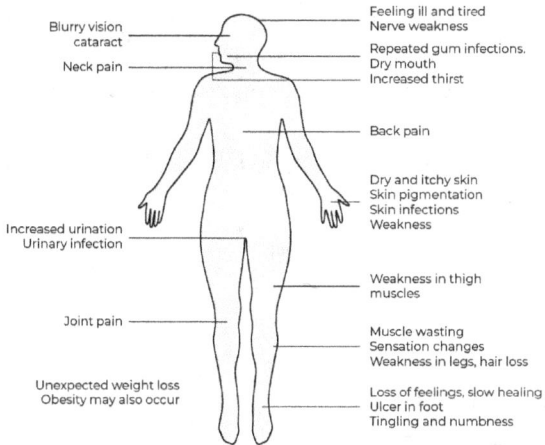

Changes in the body in diabetes mellitus

Diabetes is a commonly used term for 'Diabetes mellitus'. 'Diabetes' means a disease which is marked by excessive urination and 'mellitum' is a pharmaceutical preparation with honey as the excipient or vehicle for the drug. 'Diabetes mellitus' means passing of *excessive urine containing sugar*.

Diabetes is the condition in which the body does not properly process food for use as energy. Most of the carbohydrate food we eat is turned into glucose or sugar, for our body to use for energy. The pancreas is an organ that lies near the stomach to make insulin, a hormone that helps glucose to enter into the cells of our body and be used.

Diabetes occurs either due to the pancreas not producing enough insulin, or the cells of the body is not responding properly to the insulin produced.

There are two main types of diabetes mellitus:

- Type 1 diabetes, and
- Type 2 diabetes.

Causes of diabetes

Type 1 diabetes, also known as 'juvenile diabetes', results from the failure of the pancreas to produce enough insulin due to loss of beta cells caused by an autoimmune response. The cause of this autoimmune response is unknown.

Type 2 diabetes, also known as adult-onset diabetes. This type of diabetes results either from the reduced secretion of insulin by the beta cells of the pancrease or when insulin secretion remains normal but the body cells cannot use the secreted insulin due to the development of insulin resistance in the body cells.

Here, body pain only related to type 2 diabetes will be discussed. Any mention of 'diabetes' will be referring to Type 2 diabetes.

Classic symptoms of diabetes:

- Unintended weight loss.
- Polyuria: Increased urination.
- Polydipsia: Increased thirst.
- Polyphagia: Increased hunger.

These symptoms develop slowly and may be subtle.

Body pain associated with diabetes include pains across the entire body. Here, pains of muscles, bones and joints are discussed.

Various skeletal and/or muscular system problems arise in diabetes. The metabolic disturbances in diabetes result in changes to the bones, joints, and soft tissues. Here, the symptoms of the limbs and spine are discussed.

Common bone, muscle and joint problems include:

- Low back pain.
- Shoulder, hand, wrist, and finger pain.
- Skin problems.
- Carpal tunnel syndrome (CTS).
- Dupuytren's contracture.
- Trigger finger.

- Frozen shoulder.
- Muscle pain.
- Diabetic neuropathy.
- Diabetic foot.
- Diabetic cachexia.
- Osteoporosis.
- Osteoarthritis.

These changes ultimately manifest as the following symptoms:

- *Pain* in hands and feet due to nerve involvement.
- Pain in the body while in rest or during activity.
- *Stiff joints:* Limited joint range of movements.
- *Fracture* of bone due to increased bone fragility (osteoporosis).
- Lowering the quality of life.

Skin problems
With untreated diabetes, the skin becomes thick, tight, and waxy. These changes will contribute to the limited range of motion of the associated joints.

Hands, wrists, and fingers
The hand, wrists, and fingers are important targets for several diabetes-related complications. The mobility of the joints of the hand and wrist is reduced. The hand feels stiff and bending of the fingers towards the palm develops at advanced stages. The condition is diagnosed by the *'prayer sign'.* 'Prayer sign' is detected by the patient's inability to press their palms together completely without a gap remaining between the opposed palms and fingers.

Carpal tunnel syndrome (CTS)
CTS is often observed in diabetic patients. Diabetes-induced tissue changes cause entrapment of the *median nerve* as it passes through the wrist tunnel.

See hand pain. page:

Dupuytren's contracture
Dupuytren's contracture results from the thickening, shortening, and fibrosis of the palmar fascia. Palmar fascia is a deeply seated and thick fascia of the palm. In some cases, nodules form along the fascia. Dupuytren's contracture develops in many patients suffering from long standing diabetes.

Dupuytren's contracture. See Hand pain. Page:

Trigger finger: See hand pain. Page:

Shoulders

Diabetes can affect the shoulder in several ways. The most common effect is *adhesive capsulitis*, or *frozen shoulder*. In frozen shoulder reversible contraction of joint capsule occurs.

Frozen shoulder: page: 197.

Diabetic muscle pain

Diabetic muscle pain occurs due to infarction of muscle. This is seen in long standing diabetes mellitus. This is a type of spontaneous muscle pain and is caused by decreased blood flow to the muscles. There is no history of direct physical trauma causing the pain.

Features of diabetic muscle pain:

- Sudden and severe pain, swelling, and tenderness in the affected muscle group.
- The thigh and calf muscles are primarily affected.
- Pain may persist over several days to weeks.
- The pain resolves spontaneously over a period of a few weeks to months, in most cases.

Diabetic cachexia (amyotrophy)

Diabetic cachexia, or amyotrophy, is a nerve disorder that is a complication of long standing poorly controlled diabetes. When poorly controlled, diabetes causes inflammation in small blood vessels, causing reduced blood flow and ischemic nerve injury.

Features of diabetic *cachexia:*

- Pain, weakness, and muscle wasting present in the thighs, hips, buttocks, and legs.
- Pain can sometimes become very severe and asymmetrically distributed.

Diabetic osteoporosis (porus bone)

Diabetes increases the activity of bone destroying cells, called *osteoclast*, but decreases the activity of bone forming cells, called *osteoblasts*. This dysregulation leads to accelerated bone loss causing porus bone, osteopenia, and increased fragility of bone (osteoporosis). In addition, increased blood sugar levels inhibit bone-forming cells from building strong bones. Certain oral anti-diabetic drugs also cause bone loss as a side-effect. Finally, diabetic kidney damage results in loss of calcium which is required for building of strong bones.

See osteoporosis.page 329.

Inflammation of bone tissue and joint (osteoarthritis)

Osteoarthritis is a type of bone and joint inflammation where the cartilage covering of bones in a joint is progressively destroyed and produces pain and other symptoms. If the diabetic patient is of overweight or obese the pressure of excess bodyweight on the joint cartilage will destroy the cartilage and predisposes the weight bearing joints to the formation of *osteoarthritis*.

Osteoarthritis. Page: 318

Low back pain

Most adults suffer from low back pain and neck pain in some period of their life time. Patients with diabetes have a higher incidence of suffering from low back pain and neck pain.

The spinal discs have no blood vessels of their own and have to rely on the vessels of the vertebral bones to receive nutrients. In poorly controlled diabetes, the blood vessels are narrowed, oxygen and nutrient supply to the discs are reduced, causing the discs to degenerate and to become inflammed, causing pain. Diabetes also causes a reduction of blood and nutrition flow to the muscles causing muscle injury, cartilage damage by inflammation, and other tissue damage, such as degeneration of intervertebral disc and consequently spinal canal stenosis. All these will cause low back pain and neck pain.

See low back pain. Page: 277.

BODY PAIN AND PAIN RELIEF

Nerve injury (diabetic neuropathy)

Diabetic neuropathy is a type of nerve damage that occurs with poorly controlled diabetes for many years. While high blood sugar can injure nerves throughout the body, diabetic neuropathy most often damages nerves in the legs, feet, and hands. This type of neuropathy is also called *distal symmetric peripheral neuropathy* and is the most common type of diabetic neuropathy.

Features of diabetic neuropathy:

- Gradual onset of numbness, prickling or tingling and burning sensation in the feet and hands, which can spread upward into the legs and arms.
- Sharp, jabbing, throbbing, or burning pain in the regions.
- Extreme sensitivity to touch.
- Inability to sense temperature and pain.
- *Pain* and *burning* sensation in feet when they are under a blanket.
- Bone and joint pain.
- Muscle *weakness* in the legs and arms.
- Feeling as if *wearing gloves* or *socks* in the hands and feet.
- Lack of coordination, and frequent falling.
- Loss of control of *defecation* and *urination*.
- Chronic constipation.
- *Sexual* dysfunction.
- Abnormally *low* blood pressure.
- Serious *foot* problems, such as ulcers and infections.

Diabetes commonly affects the bone and muscle systems, resulting in pain in the body and other significant morbidity. These manifestations may go unrecognized for many months or years. However, pain management and management of many of these complications to varying degrees resulting in improvements in quality of life and more independence in activities of daily living is possible.

Home remedies for diabetic pain:

- Slowing the progression of diabetes by consistently keeping blood sugar level within a target range. Blood sugar levels may need to be individualized.
- OTC pain relieving drugs may be used initially for pain relief, but advice from physician is necessary.
- Physician advice must be taken for management of complications.
- Healthy food choices, like lean protein, non-starchy vegetables (chart), good fats (chart), and complex carbohydrates (chart).

- Warm water baths.
- Remaining active: walking, swimming, jogging, cycling etc.
- Activities of daily living must be continued.
- Short frequent walks, use of stationary bike to improve blood flow.
- Cessation of smoking.
- Use of splints, braces, walking shoes, and other aids according to the advices of the physician.
- Exercises may be selected according to the advice of physiotherapists and physicians.
- Sleeping position and sitting position must be adjusted.
- Food supplements like vitamin D, vitamin B-complex, vitamin B12, vitamin C etc. may be taken.
- Specific treatment for specific complications are advised.

When to seek medical advice:

Treatment for diabetes-related health problems are more effective if it is started early. So, medical advice should be taken as early as possible.

- To be able to control diabetes with high blood sugar levels.
- When pain is not relieved by home remedies.
- Features of infection, such as fever.
- Skin infections and cuts in the skin which do not heal.
- Repeated urinary and vaginal infections.
- Pain, numbness, weakness or tingling, especially in the hands, feet, arms, or legs. Even it seems insignificant, these feelings can be a sign of early nerve damage.
- Feeling of lightheadedness after standing from a seated position.
- Constipation.
- Troubles with vision.
- Sexual problems.

Diabetic foot

In long standing diabetes, almost all tissues in the body are affected. It is due to prolonged period of high blood sugar levels. Foot is also affected like many other tissues in the body. Foot problems occur due to involvement of nervous tissue and blood vessels.

Diabetes cause nerve damage and it leads to numbness in the feet and patient cannot feel sensation. The condition also makes it difficult to feel rubbing of shoes in the feet, irritation, soreness or infection on the foot.

This lack of sensation can lead to an increased risk of cuts, sores and blisters. These can ultimately form ulcers and even gangrene.

Blood vessels of hand and feet are also affected by long standing diabetes. Fats are deposited in these vessels and block the vessels, reducing blood flow to the hands and feet. Reduced blood flow can lead to pain, infection, ulcers and wounds that heal slowly.

Features of diabetic foot:
- Loss of feeling, Tingling and numbness in the foot.
- Painful tingling in the leg and foot.
- Discoloration of skin.
- Reduced temperature in the leg.
- Swelling in the foot and ankle.
- Blister and ulcer formation without pain.
- Wounds with or without drainage.
- Staining on socks.
- Red streaks formation in leg.
- Fever, chills.
- Corns or calluses formation.
- Dry or cracked skin around the heel.

Unfortunately, diabetes-related foot pain can not be cured. Proper management of complications of diabetes only prevent it from getting worse.

Home remedies and prevention for diabetic foot:
- Selfbody-care.
- Strictly control of diabetes.
- Use of proper fitting footwear. Footwear should be closed-toed. Avoid wearing sandals and walking bare-footed even in the living room.
- Feet should be checked everyday for sores, blisters, redness and calluses.
- Feet should be washed everyday in warm water using a mild soap and made dry especially the area between the toes before using socks.
- Feet should be kept as clean as face.
- Use of OTC pain relievers.

- Regular physical exercise is adviced.
- Body weight should be controlled.
- Healthy and balanced diet.chart
- Smoking should be avoided.
- Toenail should be trimmed once a week. Trimming done with a nail clipper straight accross. It should not be made round off the corners of toenails or cut down on the sides of the nails.
- Always wear socks or stockings. Socks and stockings should fit well and have soft elastic. If feet get cold, wear socks at night.
- If foot deformity is present, proper sized footwear should be choosed.
- Always check the inside of shoes to make sure that no objects are left inside.
- Feet should be protected from heat and cold.
- When in sitting position, feet can be put up, wiggle the toes and the ankles are moved several times a day.
- Never to sit in cross leg position for long periods.
- Thorough foot examination by diabetes doctor once a year.
- At every 2-3 months, attend a foot doctor, even if no foot problem is present.

Complications of diabetic foot:

- Skin and bone infections.
- Abscess formation in the foot.
- Gangrene formation in toes or sole of foot.
- Deformities in the foot.

When to seek medical advice:

- Uncontrolled diabetes.
- Temperature changes in the foot.
- Swelling in foot and/or ankle.
- Ulcer in the foot which does not heal.
- Pain or tingling in the foot or ankles.
- Ingrowing toe nails.
- Dry, cracked skin on the heels.
- Signs of infection in the foot.

Ear Pain (Earache)

The ear is the avenue to the heart'

- VOLTAIRE.

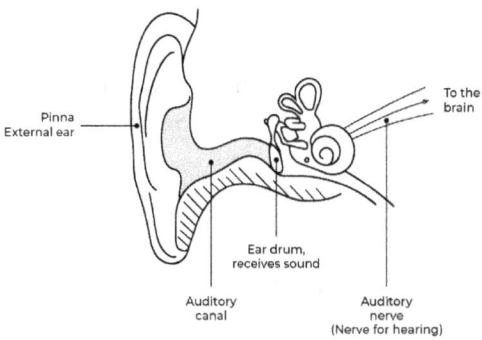

Parts of ear

Ear and parts of ear:

Ear is the organ of hearing and organ of balance.

Ear is devided into three parts: External, middle and inner ears.

External and middle ears function in transmiossion of sound. Inner ear functions as organ of balance.

External ear consists of outer visible part called pinna. It catches sound wave and amplify the sound and transmits through the ear canal to the eardrum.

Ear drum

Ear drum is also called *tympanic membrane*. When sound waves reach the tympanic membrane they cause it to vibrate. These vibrating signals are converted to an electrical signal and reaches the brain to hear the sound. Ear receives sound and finally, we hear by the brain.

Ear wax

Ear wax is a waxy and sticky substance secreted in the ear canal. Earwax trapes dust, bacteria and other germs and foreign particles that could damage ear drum.

Ear pain

Ear pain or earache is a common problem that generally occurs in children, but can also occur in adults. The majority of earache cases are not serious, but rarely it may be a serious problem. An earache may affect one or both ears, but most earaches are present only in one ear. The pain may be constant or it can come and go intermittently. Earache may be dull, sharp, or burning.

Common causes of ear pain:

- Common cold and sinus infection.
- Earwax or a foreign body in the ear.
- Water trapped in the ear.
- Ear infections.
- Tear of the eardrum.
- Infection in the throat (sore throat).
- Teeth infections.
- Jaw and jaw joint problems.
- Inflammation of the jaw joints.
- Barotrauma: Altitude pressure changes in the ear, when flying on an aircraft and causes trauma.
- Tonsil infections.
- Skin diseases in the ear canal.
- Tumor and cancer of the ear.

Features that can accompany ear pain:

Fever.
- Foul smelling discharge from the ear.
- Hearing loss, or muffled hearing.
- Sense of fullness in the ear.

Ear Pain (Earache)

- Headache.
- Jaw pain, difficulty in chewing, popping and clicking during jaw movement.
- Sleep disturbances.
- Loss of appetite.
- Loss of body balance.

Ear infection

Infection of the deeper part of the ear is common in children.

Common features of ear infection:

- Ear pain, especially when lying down.
- Pulling or tugging the ear lobe.
- Trouble hearing. Loss of balance.
- Drainage of pus or fluid from the ear.
- High fever. Headache.
- Loss of appetite.

Home remedies and prevention of ear pain:

- Cold and heat compression to the ear.
- Keep the ear dry.
- Avoid dust and allergens which can trigger allergic reactions in the body.
- Avoid smoking.
- Upright sitting will help to relieve ear pressure.
- Upright sleeping will relieve pressure on the eardrum, use of an extra pillow is beneficial.
- Sleeping with the affected ear raised instead of faced down on the pillow.
- Never introduce foreign objects in the ear.
- OTC pain relievers and/or ear drops may be used.
- Neck movement exercises may help.
- Gum chewing will help to relieve pressure within the ear.
- Olive oil may be used in the ear to soften earwax.

Foods that improve hearing functions:

- Bananas, Ginger, Garlic. Dark chocolate.
- Pumpkin seeds, flax seeds and nuts.
- Whole grains, Legumes, Spinach, kale
- Salmon. Avocado. Spinach. Kale. legumes.

BODY PAIN AND PAIN RELIEF

When to seek medical advice:

- Ear pain with fever and chills.
- Severe headache.
- Severe ear pain.
- Increased pain when wiggling the ear lobe.
- Nose blowing causes ear pain.
- Swelling around the ear.
- Blood or pus coming from the ear.
- Sudden hearing loss.
- Change in hearing or abnormal sound in the ear.
- Ringing in the ear.
- Dizziness. Vertigo.
- Drooping of facial muscle, generally on one side of the face.
- Feeling of something stuck in the ear.

Eye Pain

'The eye is the jewel of the body'

- DAVID THOREAU

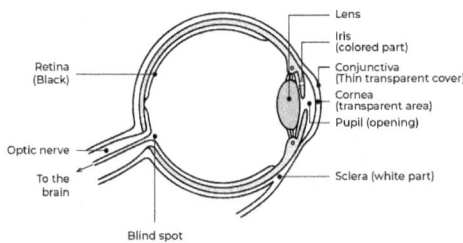

Parts of eye

The eye is the organ of sight. There are many parts of the eye. The main parts include:

Eyeball with some eye muscles and fatty tissues attached with the eyeball, and Eye lid.

Eyeball
Eyeball is a sphere like body containing sense receptors for vision and is constructed much like a simple camera. Much of the eyeball is filled with a transparent gel-like material, called vitreous humour. Vitreous humour helps to maintain the spheroidal shape of the eyeball.

BODY PAIN AND PAIN RELIEF

Parts of the eyeball:
The eyeball is composed of manny structures. Some important structures are discussed here.

- *Cornea:* The transparent area that is the front window of the eye. It transmits and focuses light into the eye.
- *Sclera:* The white area.
- *Iris:* Colored part of the eye.
- *Pupil:* The dark aperture in the iris that helps to regulate the amount of light that enters the eye.
- *Conjunctiva:* A thin membrane which covers the front part of eye ball.
- *Lens:* The transparent structure inside the eye that focuses light rays onto the retina.
- *Retina:* The nerve layer that lines the back of the eye. It senses light and creates impulses that travel through the optic nerve to the brain.
- *Eyelid:* The skin that opens and closes the eye.
- Eyelid functions:
    o Provides mechanical and anti-bacterial protection to the cornea by blinking reflexively.
    o Disperses the tear film across the eyeball surface giving lubrication and comfort.
    o Removes debris from the eyeball surface.
- *Eye muscles:* There are manny eye muscles attached with the eyeball. They control the movements of the eyeball.

Diseases and conditions that involve any of the above structures of the eye or the tissues around the eye can cause eye pain. Other types of pain associated with other areas of the body may also be felt in the eye area.

Common causes of eye pain:

- *Foreign body* in the eye.
- *Injury* to the eye.
- A blunt or sharp *trauma* or burn.
- *Infection* and inflammation of any component of eye.
- *Allergy* and irritation of the eye.
- *Dry eyes* due to decreased production of tears.
- *Refraction* problems of the lens that strain the eye.
- Problems with the *muscles* which move the eye ball.
- Problems with the *nerves* required for vision or eye movements.
- *Glaucoma:* Increase in pressure within the eyeball.

- *Cataract:* An opacity of the lens of the eye.
- *Neck pain* causing eye pain.
- Severe *headache*, cluster headache causes eye pain.

Eye pain may be associated with the following symptoms:

- Pain in one or both eyes.
- Pain in or around the eye area.
- Redness of eye.
- Double vision. Partial or complete loss of vision.
- Headache. Nausea and vomiting.
- Fever.
- Extreme sensitivity to light.
- Pain on movement of the eye.
- Feeling of flashes of light in front of eye.

Patient must seek medical advice immediately if any of the following warning signs for eye health is present:

- Severe eye pain. Double vision.
- Frequent change in visual clarity.
- Seeing distorted images.
- Veil obstructing the vision.
- Sudden loss of vision.
- Wavy or crooked appearance to straight lines.
- Swelling around the eyes.
- Seeing floaters, small objects that move around the eye field of vision.
- Flashes in the eye field of vision.
- Blind spots, dark spots in the centre of vision or around the edges of objects.
- Reduced peripheral vision and tunnel vision.
- Scratchy pain on the eye surface.
- Dryness of the eye with itching or burning.

Home care and tips for good eye health:

- Control of diabetes and high blood pressure.
- Maintaining a healthy body weight. chart
- Eating a healthy and balanced diet. chart
- Hands must be clean when touching the area around the eyes. Avoid touching the eyes frequently.

BODY PAIN AND PAIN RELIEF

- Blink frequently to help lubricate the eye surface and keep the eye healthy.
- Avoid sharing make-up sets or other eye products that could spread germs.
- Avoid smoking.
- Wear sunglasses during outdoor activities.
- Protective eye wear should always be used when performing any activity where debris could easily get into the eyes.
- Wearing protective eye gear when participating in sports, hobbies, home projects, or work-related activities.
- Eyes should be protected from computer monitor-related eye strain by looking away every 20 minutes at something 20 feet away, for 20 seconds. This will reduce eye strain and improve the eye's ability to focus. During prolonged sitting, stand up from chair every hour and take a one minute break.
- The computer screen should not be brighter than the surrounding light. Always sit away from the window to minimize glare. Glaring makes the eyes work harder and thus increases strain on the eyes.
- Care should be taken when performing activities such as putting on make-up or contact lenses to prevent eye injury.
- Regular eye examination can help to detect any problem that may be present and is necessary to make correct diagnosis and get appropriate treatment.
- Visit an eye doctor every year.

Good foods for healthy eyesight:

- Plenty of water intake to keep the body hydrated. chart
- Foods rich in anti-oxidants and omega-3 fatty acids. chart
- Food supplements: Zinc, Copper, Vitamin A, B, C, E, Beta carotene, Zeaxanthin, Lutein.
- Magnesium-rich foods: chart
- Green-tea. chart.
- Fresh fruits and vegetables.
- Retinol-rich foods: milk, liver, cheese, butter.
- Foods rich in carotenoids (Yellow and orange colored fruits): carrot, sweet potatoes, tomatoes, pumpkin, kale, apricots.
- Fresh oily fish: Tuna, Salmon, Trout, Mackrel, Sardins.
- Nuts and legumes.
- Seeds: Chia seeds, Flax seeds, Hemp seeds.

- Citrus fruits: Lemons, Oranges, Grapefruits.
- Leafy green vegetables: Spinach, Kale, Collard greens.
- Foods rach in vitamin A and betacarotene: Carrots, sweet potatoes.
- Beef contains Zinc which delays age-related sight loss.
- Eggs contain lutein and zeaxanthin and delay age-related sight loss.
- Avoid: caffeine, sugar, alcohol.

When to seek medical advice:

- Eye trauma.
- Chemical burning of the eye area.
- Foreign body in the eye.
- Swelling and redness around the eyes.
- Red eyes.
- Water, pus or blood discharge from the eye.
- Eye pain and fever.
- Eye pain and history of glaucoma in the family.
- Severe eye pain with headache, nausea and vomiting.
- Crossed eyes, where one eye is turned in a direction different from the other eye.
- Eye pain and light sensitivity.
- Seeing halos, colored circles around lights.
- Hazy or blurred vision and eye pain.
- A dark spot in the centre of field of vision.
- Pain while moving the eyes.
- Inability to keep the eye open or to close an eyelid.
- Difficulty in focusing on near or distant objects.
- Bump on the skin of the eyelids.

Some common problems in the eye.

Ulcer in the cornea

The cornea is the clear, transparent dome-shaped tissue on the frontal area of the eyeball. It covers the iris and the pupil, the opening in the iris. A corneal ulcer is a defect in the surface lining of the cornea and it is an open sore on the cornea. Corneal ulcer is usually caused by an infection.

Causes of corneal ulcer:

- Infection in the cornea.
- Eye injury due to direct trauma or chemical injury to the cornea.
- Vitamin A deficiency.
- Dry eye due to any cause.
- Faulty use of contact lenses.

Features of corneal ulcer:

- Eye pain.
- Red eye.
- Water or pus discharge from the eye.
- Foreign body sensation in the eye.
- Blurring of vision. Reduced vision.
- Increased sensitivity to light.

When to seek medical advice:

A corneal ulcer is a medical emergency. As soon as corneal ulcer is suspected, urgent medical advice is necessary.

Glaucoma

Glaucoma is a condition of eye which is usually caused by an excess accumulation of fluid in the front part within the eyeball, which increases the pressure inside the eyeball. Glaucoma damages the nerve which connects the eye to the brain and usually develops slowly. Glaucoma can cause loss of vision if it is not diagnosed and treated early. Glaucoma usually cannot be cured, but it can be stopped from progressing.

Features of glaucoma:

- Symptomless in the beginning.
- Eye pain. Headache.
- Nausea and vomiting.
- Red eye. Painful area around the eyes.
- Seeing rings around lights.
- Vision change and blurring of vision.

Eye Pain

Home remedies for glaucoma:

- Head should be kept elevated while sleeping.
- Eating a healthy and balanced diet, including foods that benefit the eyes.
- Sip fluids frequently.
- Avoid caffeine.
- Use of eye protection.
- Regular physical exercise.
- Meditation and mind relaxation.
- Use of cannabis can lower pressure in the eye.

Foods to be avoided in glaucoma:

- Avoid high trans fatty acids, chart.
- Bakery foods: cookies, cakes, donuts.
- Fried foods. Sugar. Caffeine.

When to seek medical advice:

As soon as glaucoma is suspected, immediate medical advice is a mandatory.

Nose Pain

Accepting your nose is the first step to self love.

Nose is the prominent structure between the eyes. It has a triangular-shaped projection in the center of the face. Nose gives shape to the appearance. Functionally, nose is the part of the respiratory system.

Functions of nose:

- Nose allows the air to enter the lungs.
- Filters debris and removes dust, germs and irritants.
- Warms and moistens the air and prevents them from drying out.
- Nose is the body's primary organ of smell. It takes part in sense of smell.

Nose pain is a burning sensation in the nostrils with many other associated symptoms and is very distressing. There are many causes of nose pain, and the pain may also occur in the forehead, around the eyes, and/or on the face as a whole.

Causes of nose pain:

- Common cold.
- Inflammation and infection of sinuses.
- Physical trauma to the nose. Broken nose.
- Rhinitis: Allergy in the nasal passages.
- Nasal obstruction:
    - Nasal polyp. Nasal tumor.
    - Abnormality in the nasal passage.
    - Foreign body in the nose.
- Insect bite.

Features associated with nasal pain:

- Nasal discharge may be watery or thick and yellow in color.
- Sneezing.

- Blocked nose, or difficulty in breathing through the nose.
- Itching in the nose, nasal bridge, face and/or eyes.
- Itching and pain in the throat.
- Pain and swelling around the eyes, cheeks, nose, and forehead.
- Headache due to swelling and pressure in the sinuses.
- Stiff neck.
- Persistent cough that may become worse when lying down or after getting up from lying down.
- Sleep disturbance.
- Reduced sense of smell and taste.
- Bad breath. Foul smell in breath.
- Decreased appetite.
- Weakness and fatigue.
- Changes to vision.
- Snoring.
- Fever.
- Bleeding from the nose, in rare cases.

Home remedies for the common cold:

- Steam inhalation.
- Use of a humidifier.
- Maintaining proper hydration by drinking plenty of warm water, green tea, ginger tea, fruit juice etc.
- OTC pain relievers. Anti-histamines.
- Warm compression over the nose and cheeks.
- Vitamin C and zinc supplementation. chart.
- Eating carrots, flax seeds, garlic, ginger, and onions.
- Yoga and meditation.

Avoid:

- Dairy products. Spicy, processed or fried foods.
- Caffeine.

When to seek medical advice for common cold:

- Symptoms last longer than one week.
- Swelling and redness around the eyes.
- Fever higher than 100.4°F.
- Color change of nasal discharge, greenish nasal discharge.

- Intense headache.
- Change in vision, double vision.
- Loss of smell function.
- Headache and stiff neck.
- Sleep disturbance. Confusion.
- Activities of daily life are disturbed.
- Symptoms that are getting worse day by day.
- Symptoms are not improved by OTC medications.

Fibromyalgia

(Chronic pain illness)

It takes strength to tolerate the pain everyday.

Fibromyalgia is a long term disorder characterized by widespread muscle, bone and joint pain all over the body. It is accompanied by tenderness in localised areas, fatigue, sleep, memory, and mood disorders.

Fibromyalgia is a thief. It steals body, energy, health, family, friends and lastly the person you use to be.

Fibromyalgia is not considered as a mental illness, though many people with fibromyalgia also experience depression and/or anxiety. It is thought that abnormal levels of certain chemicals in the brain change the activities of the brain, spinal cord and nerves.

Fibromyalgia amplifies painful sensations by affecting the way the brain and spinal cord process painful and non-painful signals.

Fibromyalgia typically develops between the ages of 30 and 50. It can affect individuals at any age including children and elderly and occurs both in women and men. Women are more commonly affected than men. Diffuse musculoskeletal aching and stiffness at multiple sites are observed.

Causes of fibromyalgia:

The exact cause of fibromyalgia is *not* known and it may run in families through inherited genes. Fibromyalgia is triggered by a stressful event such as physical or emotional stress, major trauma, infection, or surgery. For instance, the breakdown of a relationship or the death of a loved one may trigger the condition. Overall, fibromyalgia greatly reduces quality of life. The most commonly affected parts of the body are the *neck, shoulders, back, hips, arms,* and *legs*.

BODY PAIN AND PAIN RELIEF

Fibromyalgia can interfere with a person's daily life and create difficulties for them at work or in their home. A lack of understanding from others, chronic pain, and a lack of sleep can lead to depression and anxiety. Fibromyalgia is a chronic condition and can last a lifetime. Fibromyalgia is not a progressive disease and does not cause any direct damage to the body and it is not fatal.

Features of fibromyalgia:

- Women are more commonly affected than men (7:1)
- Age of diagnosis between 30 and 50 is more common.
- Unexplained pain and tenderness in multiple areas of body. Increased sensitivity to pain.
- Pain occurs when puts pressure on the affected area (s).
- Pain and tenderness are diffuse in character.
- Muscle stiffness, twitching and cramping.
- Tingling and numbness in the hands and feet.
- Extreme tiredness and feeling of general fatigue.
- Multiple tender points in the body.
- Problems with mental processes, including problems with memory and concentration.
- Headache. Sleep disturbances.
- Irritable bowel syndrome, stomach pain, bloating.

Home remedies and prevention:

- There is *no cure* for fibromyalgia and it is a large challenge for home care providers.

Lifestyle changes may help with pain due to fibromyalgia:

- Yoga, meditation, Tai-chi, body massage.
- Flotation and spa therapy.
- Proper and sufficient sleep.
- Low-impact exercises: swimming, cycling, walking.
- Change in daily habits to maintain normal sleep pattern.
- Mind and body relaxation.
- OTC drugs: ibuprofen, naproxen, acetaminophen.
- Healthy and balanced diet. chart.
- Food supplementation: vitamin D, Magnesium. chart.

Avoid certain foods which can flare-up symptoms:

- *Gluten:* present in wheat, rye, bread, pasta, cereals.
- *Red meat.*
- Fruits and vegetables in the *nightshade family:* tomatoes, eggplant, green peppers.
- Foods containing aspartame *(artificial sweetener).*
- Foods containing sodium nitrite *(food preservative).*
- Processed sugar. Dairy products.
- Nicotine. Caffeine. Alcohol.

Stress management

- Keeping in touch with friends and family.
- Joining a support group for people with fibromyalgia.

Body massage

Body massage involves the gentle manipulation of the body to increase the range of motion of the affected joints, reduce stress, promote relaxation, and relieve pain. Massage is a well-known treatment for sore muscles and joints. Chart.

Complications of fibromyalgia:

- Pain and tenderness becomes chronic.
- Chronic headache.
- Fatigue. Anxiety/depression. Mood disorders.
- Pain become excruciatingly worse over time.

Fibromyalgia may be mistaken for the following conditions:

- Over and under activity of thyroid gland.
- Inflammatory joint diseases.
- Chronic fatigue syndrome (myalgic encephalomyelitis).
- Gluten sensitivity.
- Myofacial pain.

When to take medical advice:

- Unbearable pain.
- Home remedies are not sufficient to alleviate symptoms.
- Fibromyalgia is complicated by other body problems.

Gout and Body Pain

'Gout is a medical term for rheumatism of rich patients'

-AMBROSE BIERCE.

Gout is a *metabolic disease* and is a type of inflammatory joint disease. It is caused by excess formation and/or accumulation of *uric acid* in the blood. It is due to inability of the kidneys to excrete uric acid efficiently. Uric acid is normally removed from the body by the kidneys. Decreased excretion of uric acid is the most common cause of gout.

Build-up of uric acid in the body causes the formation of tiny sharp crystals of uric acid in and around joints, causing inflammation and pain. Any joint in the body may be affected, but most classically gout affects the joint in the base of the great toe.

Risk factors for gout:

- Family history of gout.
- Eating foods that cause a build-up of uric acid, such as red meat, offal, seafoods.
- Kidney diseases, High blood pressure.
- Uncontrolled diabetes. Obesity.
- Drinking excess alcohol.

Features of gout:

- Severe joint pain.
- Pain almost always starts suddenly and often at night. The pain is likely to be most severe within the first 4 to 24 hours after it starts.
- Many joints may be affected simultaneously.
- The affected joints become swollen and warm.
- Color change of the skin over the joint.
- Joints become very painful to touch.

BODY PAIN AND PAIN RELIEF

- Painful movements of the affected joints.
- Joint becomes stiff and range of movement is reduced.

Home remedies and prevention of gout:

- Rest and elevation of the affected joints to reduce swelling and pain.
- Plenty of water intake. Lemon water is better and proper hydration may remove excess uric acid from the body.
- Cold pack and compress is useful in severe pain. chart.
- Maintaining a healthy body weight.
- Strict control of diabetes and high blood pressure.
- Regular physical exercise to reduce stress and keep the joints supple.
- OTC pain relievers: Ibuprofen, Naproxen, Acetaminophen.
- Magnesium and vitamin C supplement. chart.
- Drinking of coffee can lower uric acid levels.
- Ginger, Turmeric, Apple cider vinegar, lemon juice, Nettle tea, Dandelion tea, and Hibiscus tea are beneficial.
- Epsom salt bath may relieve some pain.

Foods and drinks to *avoid*:

- Processed foods. Refined carbohydrates.
- Bakery foods: refined breads, Cakes, Cookies.
- All types of alcoholic beverages.
- Red meats, Organ meats like Liver, kidney, Brain, fish eggs.
- Some fishes, like Shellfish, Sardin, Herring, Mussel, Codfish, Trout, Haddock, Shrimp, Lobster.
- Kidney beans, Lentils. Yeast.
- Canned fruit juices, Sugary drinks, Soda.
- Fructose corn syrup. Honey.

Beneficial foods and drinks in gout:

- Plenty of water to remain hydrated.
- Complex carbohydrates: Whole grains, Oats, Brown rice.
- Soy products.
- Lean meat: chicken in limited quantities, salmon, eggs.
- Fresh vegetables, especially dark green vegetables, peas, mushrooms, eggplants.
- Fresh fruits: berries, citrus fruits and avocado.
- Low fat dairy products including yogurt.

- Nuts and seeds.
- Beverages: Coffee, Tea, Green tea.
- Olive oil, Flax oil, Coconut oil, Canola oil.

When to seek medical advice:

- To confirm diagnosis.
- Pain with high fever and chills.
- Features of infection in joints. See septic arthritis: page
- Severe pain in joints.
- Multiple joints are affected.
- Marked joint stiffness.
- Flare-up of gout symptoms.

Hand Pain

The *hand* is the grasping organ of the body. It is the distal part of the forelimb and is attached to the forearm at the wrist. The hand includes the wrist, the body of the hand, and the fingers.

The hand exhibits great mobility and flexibility in the digits and throughout the whole part of the hand. The hands and wrists contain many bones, joints, ligaments, tendons, nerves and blood vessels.

The hand normally has five fingers. Finger tips contain some of the densest areas of nerve endings in the body. These nerve endings are the richest source of touch sensation. Different types of nerve endings determine whether an object is rough or smooth, hot or cold, sharp or dull. Fingertips also have the greatest positioning capability of the body. The hands play an important function in body language, sign language, and calculation techniques.

The hand has a versatile range of function. Due to the hand's remarkable adaptability to functional requirements, the hand is largely responsible for the creative manifestations that characterize the human species. These functions distinguish the human species from all other known forms of life. The hand is sometimes called the man's *outer brain*.

Hand pain is often the result of a recent injury or from overusing the hand or wrist. However, persistent or recurring pain in the hand may be the sign of an underlying disease or condition.

Causes of pain in the hand and wrist:
- Hand injuries due to physical trauma.
- Inflammation, nerve damage, sprain and fractures in the hand and wrist.
- Infection in bones, joints and soft tissues.
- Generalised chronic illness in the body.
- Overuse of the hand and wrist due to long periods of typing, heavy lifting, or playing sports.

- Inflammation of the joints of the hand and wrist.
  - Rheumatoid arthritis, page
  - Osteoarthritis, page
  - Gout, page
- Ganglion or cysts around the hand.
- Trigger finger.
- Carpal tunnel syndrome.
- De Quervain's disease.
- Dupuytren's contracture.
- Osteoporosis of the bones of the hand.
- Diseases of nerves (peripheral neuropathy).
- Raynaud's phenomenon.

Finger fractures and dislocations are common types of hand injuries. Knocks, blows, and landing on the hands during a fall are common causes of hand injuries. These types of injuries to the hand can damage structures and lead to pain, swelling, bruising and other symptoms.

Overuse injuries of the hand and wrist

Repetitive movements or overuse of the hands and wrists can cause the muscles, tendons, and nerves to become painful, sore or tense. This type of pain typically results from carrying out very repetitive or high-intensity activities for a long time. Common causes of overuse injuries include typing or using a computer mouse, using tools, lifting heavy objects, and playing or training for sports.

Home remedies and prevention of overuse hand injuries:

- Rest the hand, frequent breaks while working is helpful.
- Avoid activities which provoke pain.
- Elevating the hand is beneficial if swelling is present in the wrist and hand.
- Application of hot and cold packs.
- Gentle stretching of fingers.
- OTC pain relievers: Ibuprofen, Naproxen, Acetaminophen.
- Adjustments to working and training habits can help to prevent further injury to the hand.

When to seek medical advice:

- When home remedies do not relieve pain.
- Severe, chronic, persistent and/or recurring pain.
- Range of movements of the wrist and hand are reduced.
- Pain is accompanied by tingling and numbness in the hand.
- Gradual weakness in gripping and pinching movements.
- Reduced sensation in the hand and wrist.

Hand infection

The hand can be easily injured during everyday activities. Any trauma to the hand, particularly a penetrating injury, may introduce infecting organisms to the hand and start an infection. If an infection is not properly diagnosed and treated, significant disability in the hand can result.

Features of infection in the hand and wrist:

Pain in the hand that may spread to the forearm and arm.
- Change of color of the skin of the hand and wrist.
- Swelling in the hand.
- Hand is warm and painful to touch.
- Fever.
- Activities of hand and the upper limb may be reduced or even stopped.

As soon as infection in the hand is suspected, immediate medical advice must be taken to prevent permanent disability.

Ganglion cysts

Ganglion cysts are fluid-filled lumps that can develop near joints and tendons in the hand and wrist. Ganglions may be painful and may make use of the hand and wrist difficult.

As soon as a ganglion cyst is suspected, prompt medical advice should be sought.

Trigger finger

The tendons of the fingers allow us to be able to bend and straighten the fingers. These tendons pass through the *tunnels* or *tendon sheaths* and are called as 'pulleys'.

'Trigger finger' occurs when the ring of connective tissue, called the 'tendon sheath', situated at the base of the fingers becomes swollen and tight due to inflammation and fluid collection. The swollen tendon sheath can 'catch' the tendon in the tunnel and make the movements of the tendon difficult and painful. The finger or thumb can become stuck in a bent position. Sometimes a popping sensation is felt upon trying to move the finger.

'Trigger finger' can affect any finger, and more than one finger and/or both hands may be affected. The affected finger or thumb may eventually become permanently stuck in a bent or straightened position. Trigger finger is more pronounced in the morning and can interfere with the activities of daily life.

Risk factors for trigger finger:

- More common in women. Middle and older age groups are mainly affected.
- Diabetes mellitus.
- Repetitive finger use.
- Strong and prolonged gripping.
- Pre-existing inflammatory disease of hand and fingers, such as rheumatoid arthritis, gout, or osteoarthritis.
- Thyroid gland problems.

Features of trigger finger:

- History of pain and morning stiffness in the finger joints.
- Pain on touching the palm at the base of the affected finger.
- A small nodule may develop on the palmar aspect of the base of the finger, which is painful when pressure is applied.
- A popping or clicking sensation is felt as the finger is moved.
- Finger catching or locking in a bent position, and upon trying to straighten the finger it suddenly pops straight with severe pain. It is like a trigger of a gun being pulled and released.

Home remedies and prevention of 'trigger finger':

- Application of *heat compression* to the affected area. It will reduce edema and relax the tendons and muscles.
- Rest to the affected fingers by taking a break from repetitive activities.
- Wearing a *brace* or *splint* to give rest to the hand.

- The palm and fingers may be placed in *warm* water to reduce edema and relax the tendons and muscles.
- Gentle *stretching exercise* of the fingers to increase the range of movement.
- OTC *pain relievers:* ibuprofen, naproxen, acetaminophen.
- Use of *adaptive tools* may also help.

When to seek medical advice:

- If finger joints show the features of infection:
  - Joint swelling. Fever.
  - Overlying skin of joint is red, hot, and edematous.
  - Joint is painful on touch.
- Tingling and numbness in the fingers.
- Stiffness of the joint gradually increases.
- Finger joint cannot be bent or straightened.
- Bent finger catches in bed or in clothes.

Arthritis: Joint inflammation

Joint inflammation is called arthritis. Arthritis causes pain, swelling, and stiffness in joints. The most common type of arthritis is osteoarthritis. Other common types of arthritis include rheumatoid arthritis, gouty arthritis etc.

Features of finger joint arthritis:

- Dull or burning pain in the small joints of the hands or wrists.
- Pain after heavy gripping, overuse, or repetitive motion.
- Morning pain and stiffness in the joints of the hand.
- Swelling around the joints.
- Feeling of warmth in the affected joints.
- Sensation of grinding, grating or looseness in joints.

Home remedies for finger arthritis:

There is *no cure* for rheumatoid arthritis and osteoarthritis. However, proper treatment can:
  - Slow down the progression of the disease.
  - Relieve pain and some other symptoms.
  - Preserve mobility of the joint.
- *Heat therapy:* relax muscles, reduce muscle tension and reduce pain sensitivity.
  - Soaking hands in warm water.

- Taking warm shower.
  - Applying warm compresses or *heating pads* to the inflamed and painful hands.
  - A *moist heat* pad may also be used.
  - Treating hand with a paraffin *wax bath*.
  - *Warm dress* is beneficial.
- *Cold therapy:* Severe and acute pain in the finger may be relieved to some extent. Cold packs can numb sore hands and reduce inflammation and swelling.
- *OTC pain relievers:* Ibuprofen, Naproxen, Acetaminophen.
- *Simple finger exercises:* Finger and hand exercises can strengthen the hand muscles. Exercises increase blood flow to the tissues surrounding the joint. This blood flow keeps the tissues healthy and strong and prevents further breakdown of cartilage. Stronger muscles will also increase efficiency of hand movements and functions.

Common exercises include:

- Repeated making and opening of the fists.
- Bending and straightening of the fingers.
- Thumb bends.
- Making of a 'C' or an 'O' with the fingers
- Finger lifting. Wrist bends.
- Squeezing a rubber ball.
- Applications of finger splints: Use of hand and finger splints reduce pain and swelling and improve joint mobility. Compression gloves may also be used.
- Massage: chart
- Eating a healthy and balanced diet. chart
- Foods beneficial for arthritis. See
- Meditations and mindfulness.

Carpal tunnel syndrome (CTS)

Carpal tunnel syndrome occurs when the median nerve, which passes through the wrist tunnel, becomes compressed due to inflammation and edema of the soft tissues around the nerve. Symptoms can start gradually and are often worsen at night.

Risk factors for CTS:

- Pre-existing inflammatory diseases of joints (arthritis).
- Diabetes mellitus. High blood pressure.
- Pregnancy. High salt intake.
- Smoking. Sedentary lifestyle.

Features of carpal tunnel syndrome:

- Pain or prickling sensation and numbness in the hand and fingers. Pain starts gradually over time.
- Pain is throbbing in character and occurs when the wrist and fingers are moved.
- Discomfort becomes worse at night and upon keeping the wrist in an overextended position (bending backwards) for too long time.
- Tingling and numbness in the hand, fingers and arm.
- Decreased grip strength and weakness in the hand, often dropping objects from the hand.
- Precise movements of fingers are affected.
- Difficulty in grasping small objects.
- Wasting of muscles at the base of the thumb.
- Difficulties in writing and typing.

Home remedies and prevention of carpal tunnel syndrome:

- Avoid repetitive tasks requiring the wrist.
- Take breaks between activities.
- Avoid using a firm grip.
- Avoid bending the wrist. Keep the wrist in neutral position as much as possible.
- The wrist and palm should be kept warm. Wearing fingerless gloves is helpful.
- 'Making and opening a fist' exercise whenever possible will help to relieve pressure on the wrist.
- Elevate the hand and wrist whenever possible.
- OTC pain relievers and topical cream may be used.

When to seek medical advice:

- If home treatment for 2 weeks does not relieve pain and symptoms become more severe.

- Tingling, numbness, and weakness in the fingers has gradually increased, ultimately progressing to little or no feeling in the fingers.
- Simple hand movements are difficult.
- Normal activities of daily life are difficult.
- Intermittent dropping of objects from the hand.
- Pain in the hand disturbs normal sleep.

Dupuytren's contracture

Dupuytren's contracture results from the thickening, shortening, and fibrosis of the palmar fascia. The palmar fascia is the deeply seated, thick sheath of tissue in the palm. Sometimes nodules are formed along the fascia. Dupuytren's contracture develops in many patients suffering from long standing diabetes.

Risk factors for Dupuytren's contracture:

- Most common in older adults and more common among males.
- Family history of 'Dupuytren's contracture'.
- Medications for epilepsy will enhance.
- Diabetes mellitus.
- Smoking and alcohol consumption.

Features of Dupuytren's contracture:

Deformity develops over several years.
- Both hands may be affected.
- Knots of tissue form under the skin.
- Knots gradually form thick cords that can pull one or more fingers into a bent position towards the palm.
- The affected fingers cannot be straightened completely.
- The bent finger can complicate everyday activities like placing hand in the pockets, putting on gloves, or shaking hands.
- Mainly affects the two fingers farthest from the thumb.
- Thumb and index fingers are rarely affected.
- Same type of problems may develop in the sole of feet and penis.

Home remedies and prevention:

There is no cure for 'Dupuytren's contracture'. At home remedies can help to slow the progression of the condition.

- Protect the palm and hand by wearing hand gloves.
- Using a looser grip is beneficial. Avoid using a firm grip.

- Stretching exercises for the fingers and hand. Seek medical advice as necessary.
- Massage to the palm and hand. Benefits:chart
- Eat a healthy and balanced diet, including anti-inflammatory foods. See chart.
- Smoking and alcohol should be avoided.
- Vitamin E, Zinc, Magnesium supplementation.

Osteoporosis

Osteoporosis is the gradual loss of bone mass, causing the bones to become weak and brittle. Bones with osteoporosis become prone to fracture, particularly in the wrist and hips. Osteoporosis occurs more in females and in older adults.

Risk factors for osteoporosis: See Osteoporosis, page:319.

Features of osteoporosis in the hands and fingers:

- Weaker grip strength.
- Weak and brittle finger nails.
- Wrist fracture occurs more easily due to falls.

Home remedies and prevention of osteoporosis, page

When to seek medical advice for osteoporosis, page

De Quervain's disease (DQD)

'De Quervain's disease' is a painful wrist condition caused by the inflammation of two tendons and their tendon sheaths. These two tendons control the movements of thumb. The tendons are on the thumb side of the wrist and cause pain upon moving the thumb, turning the wrist, grasping and in making a fist and in a pinching motion. There may be swelling near the base of the thumb and the pain may radiate to the thumb or forearm. There may also be popping feeling when moving the thumb.

Risk factors for DQD:

- Women, middle-aged and older adults are mainly affected.
- Pregnancy.
- Repetitive thumb and wrist movements.
- Caring for a child: repeated lifting a baby puts strain on the thumbs, as such this condition is also called 'mommy thumb'.

BODY PAIN AND PAIN RELIEF

- Pre-existing inflammatory disease in the body, such as rheumatoid arthritis, gout, etc.
- Diabetes mellitus.

Home remedies and prevention of DQD:

- Heat and cold compression at the painful site and wrist.
- Avoiding repetitive movements of the wrist and thumb.
- Avoid overuse of the wrist.
- Wrist and finger actions should be changed to reduce stress on the wrist.
- Take frequent breaks during activities to rest the wrist.
- Avoid repetitive grasping and pinching.
- Avoid direct blows to the thumb.
- Bracing or splinting the thumb and wrist will help. Seek medical advice as necessary.
- OTC pain relievers: ibuprofen, naproxen, acetaminophen.

When to seek medical advice:

- If the condition does not respond to home treatment and/or the condition gradually worsens.
- Movements of the thumb make the condition worse.
- Range of movement of the thumb is gradually reduced.
- Gradually increased weakness of thumb movements.
- Shows features of infection:
    - Skin over the wrist becomes red.
    - Wrist swelling.
    - Fever.
    - Pain on touching and pressing the wrist.

Degeneration of the peripheral nerve (peripheral neuropathy)

The peripheral nerves form a network of 43 pairs of motor and sensory nerves. These nerves connect the brain and spinal cord to the entire body, including the muscles, skin, and internal organs. The peripheral nerves control the functions of sensation, movement and motor coordination and can be damaged easily.

Peripheral neuropathy is a condition resulting from damage to the peripheral nerves due to disease and/or deficiencies. Peripheral neuropathy frequently starts in the hands and feet, but other parts of the body may also be affected.

Risk factors for peripheral neuropathy:

- Traumatic injury to the nerve.
- Nerve compression.
- Infection of the nerve by virus, bacteria or other organisms.
- Metabolic causes: Diabetes mellitus, thyroid problems.
- Genetic causes.
- Exposure to toxins, like lead or mercury.
- Poor nutrition, including deficiency of certain vitamins and minerals.
- Anti-cancer drugs.
- Chronic diseases: kidney failure, liver failure, thyroid diseases, rheumatoid arthritis.

Features of peripheral neuropathy:

- Gradual onset of prickling, tingling, and numbness in the hands.
- Sharp jabbing, throbbing, burning, and stabbing pain in hands which can be described as lightening-like pain.
- A feeling of weakness, heaviness, and locking in the arms and legs.
- Extreme sensitivity to touch in the area.
- Generalized muscular weakness.
- Pain in the feet and hand when they are placed under a blanket. Feeling as if tight gloves or socks are worn.
- Paralysis, if motor nerves are severely affected.
- Heat intolerance.
- Hot and cold sensitivity in the area.

Home remedies and prevention:

- Regular physical exercise will improve blood supply to the limbs and improve muscle tone and strength.
- Eating a healthy and balanced diet.
- Maintaining a healthy body weight.
- Strict control of diabetes.
- Dietary changes:
  - High fiber foods. chart.
  - Anti-oxidant rich foods. chart
  - Omega-3 fatty acid rich foods. chart
  - Vitamin supplementation: Vitamin B_1, B_6, B_9, B_{12}.

Vitamin B_1, B_6, B_{12}: relieves neuropathic pain.

Vitamin B_9, B_{12}: maintains protective coating of nerves.

- o Magnesium and calcium supplementation.
- Avoid smoking.
- Meditation and mental relaxation.

When to seek medical advice:

- Unusual tingling, numbness, and weakness in hands and feet.
- Pain and burning sensation in the hands and feet.
- Symptoms suddenly becoming worse.
- Development of sores in the hands and feet.
- Features of infection present.
- Pain and other symptoms spread to another area of the body.
- Difficulty in maintaining activities of daily life.

Hand-arm vibration syndrome

Hand-arm vibration syndrome is caused by repeated minor injuries to the small nerves and blood vessels in the fingers. This type of injury typically affects people who have regularly used vibrating tools and machinery over a long period of time. Such tools include pneumatic drills, power drills, and chainsaws. Early symptoms include a loss of feeling, numbness, and sensations of pins and needles in the fingers. Symptoms can often be mild, only affecting the finger tips, however numbness may affect the whole finger. For some people doing up buttons and picking up small objects like coins will be difficult. Hand-arm vibration syndrome can lead to Raynaud's phenomenon.

Raynaud's phenomenon

Raynaud's phenomenon is a condition in which the blood vessels in the fingers or toes temporarily narrow. It often occurs in response to cold temperatures or stress. During a flare-up, blood flow to the hands becomes severely reduced. This may cause the skin of the fingers to lighten or become blue and the fingers may become numb or painful. When the blood flow begins to return, the hands may appear red or purple. The length of these attacks can vary from less than a minute to several hours.

Common symptoms associated with general hand pain:

- Numbness in the hand(s).
- Trouble in gripping objects with the hand(s).
- A feeling of 'pins and needles' in the fingers.

- Swelling in the fingers.
- Burning or tingling in the fingers, especially the thumb, index, and middle fingers.

Home remedies for general hand pain:

- Avoidance of causative factors.
- Lifestyle changes.
- Exercises to keep the hand physically active.
- Stretching of the hand and fingers.
- Applications of heat and cold compression, hot compress for stiffness and cold compress for swelling.
- OTC pain medication.
- Use of splint to stabilize joints and rest the hand.

Prevention of general hand pain:

- Avoid work and movements that worsen the pain.
- Avoid overuse of the hand.
- Rest the hand, use splints when necessary.
- Heat and cold compression.
- Stretching exercises of the wrist, hand, and fingers.
- Use of custom-made tools for daily activities.
- Modifying job requirements.
- Typical activities of daily life should be continued as much as possible.
- OTC pain relievers: acetaminophen, naproxen, ibuprofen.

Lifestyle changes for chronic hand pain:

Lifestyle changes can positively impact chronic hand pain to a great extent.

Benefits include:

- Reducing the demand for pain relieving drugs.
- Improving circulation and making tissues healthier.
- Decreasing the rate of joint and other tissue damage.
- Improving joint range of movement.
- Improving skills while working.

Common lifestyle changes for chronic hand pain include:

- Frequently adjusting body position. The patient should determine the best body position which eases hand pain.

BODY PAIN AND PAIN RELIEF

- While resting, the shoulders and hands should be kept relaxed.
- Determine the most comfortable position for work and other activities.
- Avoid exposure to extreme cold and hot temperatures.
- Protective gear and supportive gloves may be used for repetitive tasks and use of certain equipment.
- Reduce the speed and duration of fine hand movement activities that cause chronic hand pain, such as typing, writing, or sewing.
- Avoid keeping the hand stationary for long periods. Hand position should be changed frequently.
- While grasping an object, use the entire hand, rather than just the thumb and index finger. Using the entire hand spreads the weight of the object and reduces stress on the wrist.
- Where possible, use tools to assist in some tasks.

Use of a computer keyboard

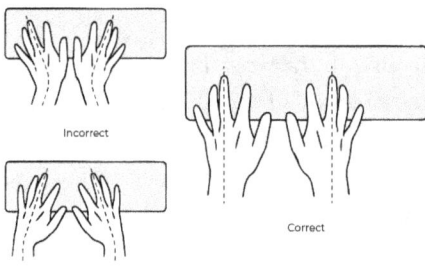

When using a laptop computer, use of an external keyboard is ideal. The laptop screen should be 25 inches away from the eyes. Place the keyboard just below elbow level while in a seated position. Elbows should be kept at an open angle between 90-110° and hanging close to the body. This position relaxes the forearms and shoulders. The keyboard should be kept flat on the desk, or with a slight and gentle negative slope. The wrists should be kept in a straight position, neither bent upwards or downwards. Resting the wrists on the desk while the fingers are on the keyboard should be avoided, as this posture may put pressure on the wrist and may hamper blood supply to the wrist, hand, and fingers. While using a keyboard, the feet should be flat on the floor, or a footrest while seated may be used.

Change wrist, hand, and forearm posture frequently while working. Forearm and wrist stretching will help avoid pain while typing. While typing, the fingers should be kept relaxed. Typing lightly will prevent the fingers from getting tired, which will help avoid pain.

Use of a computer mouse

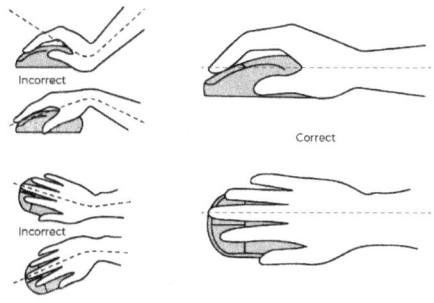

If possible, use of a vertical mouse, ergonomic mouse or roller mouse is better than a traditional mouse. A vertical mouse maintains the hand in a handshake position, which is a more natural hand position, helping to prevent wrist pain. The mouse should be held loosely in the hand and a firm grip should be avoided. The wrist and forearm should not rest on the mousing surface, as it may hamper blood flow through the wrist. The arm should be kept hanging close to the side of the trunk, with the elbow bent at 90°.

Take frequent breaks and reduce mouse speed. An improperly shaped mouse and improper mouse use can give rise to 'mouse arm syndrome', causing pain in the hand, wrist, elbow, and shoulder.

BODY PAIN AND PAIN RELIEF

When to seek medical advice for general hand pain:
- Activities of daily life cannot be maintained.
- New and sudden onset of pain.
- Pain suddenly worsens.
- Hand pain causes loss in working hours.
- Pain due to physical trauma.
- OTC pain medications do not relieve pain.

Finger Pain

Finger pain is common and nearly everyone has had finger pain at some time in their life. Finger pain includes any kind of discomfort and pain in the tissues or joints of the fingers. Finger pain is often the result of minor injuries that can be treated at home with rest and immobilization. However, severe, worsening, or recurring pain may be the sign of a more serious injury or an underlying disease. Individuals should seek medical advice for finger pain or symptoms that impact daily activities and/or if they suspect a fracture, dislocation, or wound infection.

The finger is made up of bones, muscles, blood vessels, nerves, and skin. Each finger has 3 joints and the thumb has 2 joints. A joint is made up of bones, cartilage, capsule, ligaments, tendons, bursas, and synovial membrane. Bursas are fluid-filled sacs that cushion the tendons and ligaments. The synovial membrane forms a cavity that contains synovial fluid which helps to lubricate the opposing joint surfaces.

Any of the structures in the finger can become irritated, inflamed, and painful in response to a variety of mild to serious diseases, disorders, or conditions. Trauma, infection, inflammation, tumors, and nerve compression are important causative factors.

In most cases, finger pain is not a serious condition and will resolve on its own. However, unexplained finger pain can be a sign of a more serious medical condition. Medical advice should be sought if there is ongoing or unexplained pain in the fingers.

Causes of finger pain:

There are many causes of finger pain that may be injury-related or non-traumatic.

Injury-related causes of finger pain:
- Cut to the skin of the finger.
- Fracture of finger bone. Stress fracture.

- Falling on the hand. Knocks and blows.
- Jamming the finger.
- Dislocation of a finger joint.
- Contusion or abrasion. Crush injury.
- Degloving injury: The skin and the top layer of tissue of the finger is separated from top to the end of the finger, like removing a glove from the hand.
- Laceration or blunt trauma.
- Repetitive stress injury.
- Penetrating injury.
- Sprain or strain of any finger joint.
- Splinter or other foreign body penetration.
- Overextending the fingers, or bending them too far backward.

Infectious, inflammatory, and degenerative causes of finger pain:

- *Osteoarthritis:* Age-related wear and tear on the joints.
- *Rheumatoid arthritis:* Inflammation of the finger joints.
- *Tenosynovitis or trigger finger:* Inflammation of the tendon sheath.
- *Tendonitis:* Inflammation of the tendon.
- *Bursitis:* Inflammation of the bursa sac.
- *Tumor* of any structure of the finger.
- *Cellulitis:* Invasive skin infection that spreads to the surrounding tissues.
- *Ganglion:* Benign cystic growth or swelling of synovial membrane.
- *Osteomyelitis:* Bacterial infection of the bone of the finger.
- *Septic* arthritis: Infection within the finger joint.
- *Infection* around the nail.
- *Osteoporosis:* Loss of bone tissue of the finger.
- *Muscular* dystrophy: Degeneration of muscles of the finger.

Nerve-related causes of finger pain:

- Compression of nerves in the wrist, elbow, or arm.
- Compression of nerves in the vertebral column.
- Injury to the neck causing nerve injury.
- Nerve damage due to diabetes mellitus.
- Transverse myelitis: Inflammation of the spinal cord.
- Underactive thyroid gland.
- Neuroma: Nerve tumor in the finger.
- Peripheral neuropathy: Nerve degeneration due to nutrition and vitamin deficiencies, e.g, vitamin B_1, B_2, B_6, B_{12} and vitamin C.

- Spinal cord tumor.
- Stroke.
- Traumatic injury to the spinal cord.
- Rare neurological diseases.

Other causes of finger pain:

- Reduced blood flow to the finger due to diseases of the blood vessels.
- Buerger's disease: Inflammation and clotting of arteries and veins.
- Frost bite: Extremely cold temperatures.
- Raynaud's disease: Spasm of small blood vessels of the fingers.
- Uncontrolled diabetes and hypertension.
- Some chronic diseases.

Symptoms that occur with finger pain:

Finger pain may be accompanied by many other symptoms. These additional symptoms vary depending on the underlying diseases, disorders, or conditions. Other symptoms that may occur with finger pain include:

- Swelling of the finger, fever, redness, warmth, and chills will occur when finger pain is due to a serious infection in the finger that has spread throughout the body.
- Arm or wrist pain.
- Decreased grip strength.
- Stiffness of finger joints.
- Reduced range of movement of the affected joint.
- Drainage of pus.
- Lacerations, abrasions, sores, or other lesions in the finger.
- Lumps or bumps along the finger.
- Tingling, numbness, and prickling sensation in the finger.

Serious symptoms:

Several symptoms associated with finger pain may indicate a serious condition that should be immediately evaluated in an emergency setting. These include:

- High fever (>101°F)
- Inability to move the finger, wrist, or arm.
- Partial or total amputation of finger.
- Red, warm and tender skin.
- Severe pain in the finger.
- Visible deformity of finger.

BODY PAIN AND PAIN RELIEF

Identifying different types of finger pain.

Pain due to broken finger
- History of direct trauma to the finger.
- Pain, swelling, tenderness, and deformity in the finger.
- Bruising or abrasion at the trauma site.
- Inability to move the finger.

Pain due to infection
- Pain gradually worsens.
- Swelling of the finger.
- Skin flushing or warmth.
- High fever.
- Pus or discharge from the cut or wound.
- Feeling sick.

Pain due to osteoarthritis
- More common in older adults.
- Joint close to fingertip is most commonly affected Fig:
- Previous history of joint injury may be present.
- Pain worsens with activity.
- Swelling of finger joints.
- Tenderness in the joint.
- Joint stiffness.
- Reduced range of movement of the affected joints.
- Pain worsens each day.

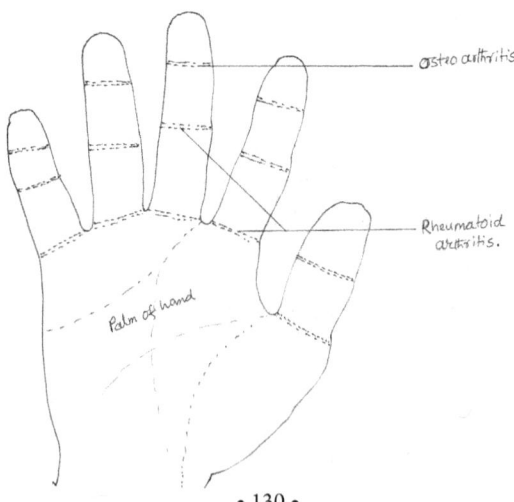

Pain due to rheumatoid arthritis
- The exact cause of rheumatoid arthritis is not known.
- Pain and stiffness in the finger that lasts for more than an hour upon waking-up in the morning or after a long period of inactivity.
- More common in women and can run in families.
- Finger joints, particularly the middle joints and joints nearer to the palm proper are more commonly affected.
- Joints are warm and painful to touch.
- Pain, swelling, stiffness, and deformity of the fingers.
- Fever.
- Numbness and prickling sensation in the finger.
- Feeling of fatigue and lack of energy.

Pain due to nerve compression in the wrist
This condition is called carpal tunnel syndrome (CTS). See hand pain 161.

Neuropathy
Pain due to nerve degeneration. See hand pain

Pain due to overuse injury
- Repeated use of hand and fingers in different industrial activities.
- Heavy hand worker.
- Use of computer mouse and keyboard for prolonged period.

Trigger finger: See hand pain, page

Pain due to lumps in the finger
- Different types of tumors of skin, soft tissues, or bone.
- Different types of arthritis.
- Infection of any component of finger.
- Trauma to the finger, even bug bites may be responsible.

To make a diagnosis, patients must know key information related to the cause of their finger pain.

These common questions include:
- Have you had a recent injury?
- What is the exact location of the pain?

BODY PAIN AND PAIN RELIEF

- Describe the pain. Is it sharp or dull, tingling or burning?
- When did pain start?
- How long does the pain last?
- Does the pain occur during or after certain activities?
- Do you have any other symptoms other than pain, such as swelling?
- What is your medical history, including past medications?
- Have had been suffering from diabetes mellitus, hypertension, or any other chronic systemic disease?
- Do you have a family history of pain which occurs without any obvious causes?

Home care for finger pain due to mild trauma:

- Any ring on the finger must be removed immediately.
- The hand and finger must be kept rested. Buddy taping the affected finger to an adjacent finger may help.
- Avoid lifting heavy objects and a tight grip.
- Elevate the hand above the level of the chest to reduce swelling.
- Apply ice to the affected area for up to 3 to 5 minutes at a time.
- OTC pain relievers: Acetaminophen, Ibuprofen, Naproxen.

When to seek medical advice:

- Hand and/or finger injury due to a trauma like a fall or crush injury.
- Infection of the finger which is marked by pain, swelling, fever, redness, and warmth. Symptoms increase day by day and activities of daily life are affected.
- Pain does not respond to home treatment for 2-3 days.
- Obvious deformity of fingers due to dislocation or fracture.
- Discoloration of the finger.
- Broken bone in the finger.
- Loss of sensation in the finger and hand.
- Sensation of pins and needles or numbness in the finger.
- Pain associated with uncontrolled diabetes.

Potential *complications* of finger pain:

There can be many complications of finger pain, that will vary depending on the underlying diseases and conditions. Some of these complications are very serious. Patients must be alert when experiencing persistent pain or other unusual symptoms related to the fingers and hands. These include:

- Chronic pain, persistence of pain, and disability.
- Finger deformity.
- Auto amputation of finger.
- Inability to perform activities of daily life.
- Spread of infection to other parts of the body.

Foot and Heel Pain

'I firmly believe that with the right footwear one can rule the world.'

—Bette Midler

Pain in the foot and heel is a common problem. The foot transmit the weight of the body to the ground. As we age, the physical shape of our foot also changes, modifying the mechanics of weight transmission. Changes to the mechanics of weight transmission will predispose to the development of foot pain.

The foot has a complicated structure consisting of 28 bones, 30 joints, Achillis' tendon and many other tendons, plantar fascia and many other fascia, ligaments, muscles, bursa, nerves, blood vessels and a special kind of skin on the bottom of the foot.

The heel is the prominence at the posterior end of the foot made up of the projection of the heel bone. The heel bone is the most posterior bone of the foot. The sole of the foot is covered by a layer of soft but tough tissue of up to 5 mm in thickness. This tissue acts as a shock absorber and stabilizes the sole.

During walking, the heel is the first part of the foot to strike the ground. The compressive forces exerted on the heel are then distributed along five rays, three in the direction of the big toe and two to the little toe. Together, these rays form the arch of the foot. The arch of the foot is optimized to distribute compressive forces across the foot over uneven surfaces. The heel thus forms the posterior point of support that, together with the balls of the large and little toes, bears the brunt of compressive loads.

The plantar fascia is a broad fibrous structure which runs from the heel bone to the heads of the forefoot bones. The plantar fascia supports the arch along the bottom of the foot. The Achilles tendon is the largest and strongest tendon in the body. It is a tough band of fibrous tissue that connects the calf muscle to the heel bone.

BODY PAIN AND PAIN RELIEF

While the bones and other soft tissues of the foot form the arch of the foot, the plantar fascia acts as a spring. The arch sustains the weight of the body and forces exerted during walking, jumping and running in such a way that we do not feel jerking during these movements. When these arches are lost, a flat foot results and repeated trauma due to movements will cause injury to the joints and other tissues of the foot, causing inflammation and pain.

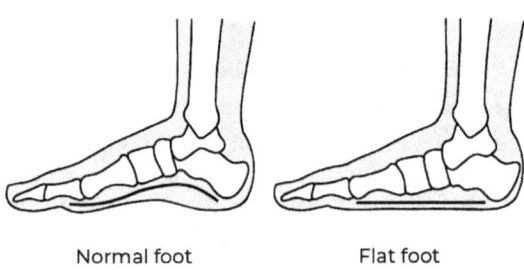

Loss of arch and flat foot.

Causes of foot and heel pain:

- Inflammation of the plantar fascia, Achilles tendon and other tendons, fascias, ligaments, bursas, and other tissues.
- Infection of bones, joints, and other tissues.
- Trauma to the foot and ankle and ankle sprain.
- Tumors of any tissue of the foot or heel.
- Corns, Calluses, and Bunions.
- Abnormal shapes of foot and heel.

Factors that aggravate foot and heel pain:

- Uncontrolled diabetes mellitus.
- Walking barefoot on hard surfaces.

- Using hard and/or ill-fitting shoes and slippers.
- Abnormal shapes of the foot and heel.
- Excess body weight.
- Unhealthy foot hygiene.

Ankle sprain

The ankle joint is a strong and stable joint that carries the weight of the body and transmits force of the weight of the body to the foot. The strong ligaments of the ankle help to stabilize the joint and prevent excessive movements. An ankle sprain is the most common ankle injury. A sprained ankle occurs when the ligaments are extended beyond their normal range of movement. When the ankle is rolled, twisted or turned in an awkward way, abnormal stretching of the tough bands of ligaments may cause tearing of the ligaments, known as an ankle sprain.

Features of a sprained ankle:

Features of an ankle sprain vary depending on the severity of the injury.

Common features include:

- *Pain* following injury to the joint that is aggravated when standing and walking.
- *Swelling* of the joint. *Bruising* over the area.
- Restricted joint range of motion.
- Ankle *instability*.
- Sound of tearing of ligaments at the time of injury.

When to seek medical advice:

As soon as an ankle sprain is suspected medical advice should be sought.

Plantar fasciitis

Inflammation of the plantar fascia is known as plantar fasciitis.

Features of plantar fasciitis:

- Stabbing pain and stiffness in the bottom of foot near the heel.
- The pain is a typical *'start-up pain'.* Pain that is worst when first getting up in the morning, or when first getting up from a period of sitting or lying position.

BODY PAIN AND PAIN RELIEF

- Localised tenderness at the inner aspect beneath the heel and sometimes in the mid foot.
- Pain is usually worse after exercise, not during exercise.

Achilles tendonitis

Inflammation of Achilles tendon is known as Achilles tendonitis.

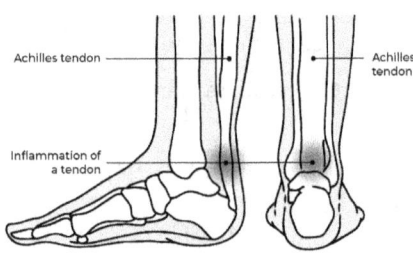

Achilles tendinitis

Features of Achilles tendonitis:
- Pain and stiffness behind the heel and along the Achilles tendon.
- Pain is marked when running fast, or when climbing stairs.
- Marked stiffness in the morning that improves with mild activity.
- Pain worsens with walking, sometimes making walking impossible.
- Tendon thickening and swelling, causing the tendon to be painful to touch that gets worse throughout the day with activities.
- The skin of the heel is warm.
- Tight calf muscles and reduced movement in turning the foot upwards toward the shin bone.
- Feeling of weakness in the leg and foot.

Joint inflammation
Features of inflammation of the joints of the foot:
- Pain in ankle joint and foot during walking and at rest.
- Swelling around the ankle joint.
- Ankle and foot stiffness.
- Deformity of the ankle joint, appearing lumpy.
- Feelings of instability and insecurity while walking.
- Tingling and numbness in the foot and toes.
- Pain upon pressing on the joint.

Septic Arthritis
Infection of the foot and ankle joints, known as septic arthritis, is not uncommon. Though there are many joints in the foot, generally a single joint is affected. Prompt diagnosis and proper treatment will reduce future complications.

Features of foot and ankle joints septic arthritis:
- Pain while walking and during joint movements.
- Swelling of the joint.
- Joint feels warm to touch.
- Fever.
- Pain on touching or pressing the joint.
- Color changes of the skin over the joint.
- Joint stiffness.

See also: Septic arthritis, Page

BODY PAIN AND PAIN RELIEF

Corns and calluses

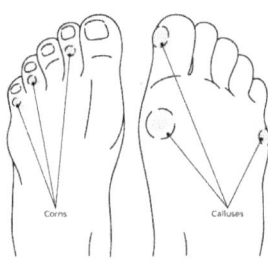

Corns and calluses are thick, hardened areas of skin on the foot, that develop when the skin tries to protect itself against prolonged rubbing and other form of irritation, friction, and pressure. Corns and calluses most often develop on the feet and toes. The hands and fingers may also be affected.

Calluses

Calluses usually develop on the weight bearing areas, such as the soles of the feet, especially under the heels or base (balls) of the toes. They can also occur on the palms, knees, elbows, and ankles due to high pressure on those areas. Calluses vary in size and shape and are generally larger and more diffuse than corns. Calluses are rarely painful. Some calluses are related to walking problems or foot abnormalities that place unusual stress on parts of the foot during walking.

Corns

Corns are smaller, round, and well defined, with a hard center surrounded by inflamed skin. Corns tend to develop on the parts of the feet that do not bear weight, such as the tops and sides of the toes and even in between the toes. Corns are caused by pressure or friction and are painful when pressed.

Causes of corns and callus formation:
- Wearing ill-fitting shoes.
- Wearing shoes without socks.
- Deformity of the foot with ill-fitting shoes.
- Features of corns and calluses:

- A thick and rough area of skin.
- A hardened and raised bump.
- Pain under the skin.
- Flaky, dry or waxy skin.
- Difficulty in grasping objects or walking.

Home remedies and prevention of corns and calluses:

- Avoid repetitive actions that cause friction.
- Wear well-fitting and comfortable shoes and socks.
- Use protective pads for areas where friction occurs.
- For a deformed foot, use shoe inserts.
- Soften the corn or callus by soaking the hand or foot in warm, soapy water and use a pumice stone to remove the dead skin from a callus or corn. Proper use of pumice stone is important. As improper use may injure the healthy skin.
- Use of moisturizing creams and ointments are beneficial.
- Wearing gloves or other protective devices.
- Use of OTC liquids or ointments that contain salicylic acid to soften the callus or corn.
- Use of OTC pads designed for corns and calluses.

When to seek medical advice:

- When the callus or corn is inflamed and very painful.
- Uncontrolled diabetes with painful corns or calluses.
- Ulcers around the corn or callus.

Ingrown toenails

Ingrown means growing inward so that a portion that is normally free becomes covered (Taber's Medical Dictionary). Ingrown toe nails are a common condition in which the corner or side of a toenail grows into the soft flesh, and the corner of the toenail which is normally free and visible becomes invisible. The big toe is most likely to be affected, but ingrowth can occur on any nail.

BODY PAIN AND PAIN RELIEF

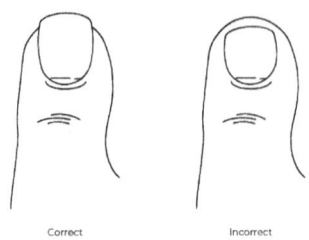

Correct   Incorrect

Trimming toenails

Causes of ingrown toenails:

- Cutting toenails too short and rounded, with corners cutback.
- Wearing ill-fitting shoes that are too tight, narrow, or flat for the feet will cause bunching of the toes and will cause the nail to curl and dig into the skin.
- Genetic predisposition to congenitally curved toenails.
- Repeated trauma to the nails.
- Athletic activities can increase the susceptibility of ingrown toenails: ballet, football, kickboxing, soccer.
- Thick nails in older adults.
- Sweaty feet and tight shoes.
- Poor posture and gait.
- Improper foot hygiene.

Features of ingrown toe nails:

- Pain and tenderness in the toes along one or both sides of the nail.
- Swelling and redness around the nails.
- Infection and pus formation.
- Overgrowth of skin around the nail.

Home remedies and prevention of ingrown toenails:

- The feet should be kept dry and as clean as the face.
- Diabetes should be strictly controlled.

- In case of infection, feet may be soaked in warm water 2-3 times daily and then well dried
- OTC pain relievers: acetaminophen, naproxen, ibuprofen.
- A tiny piece of cotton bud may be gently pushed under the corner of the nail where it is ingrown.
- Repeatedly pushing the skin away from the toenail edge with a cotton ball is helpfull.
- Use of toenail brace or plastic gutter splint. Advice from experts is required.
- Toenails should be trimmed straight across keeping the nail long enough, at least 1-2 mm beyond the tip of the flesh of the toes. Never to cut the nail rounded and cutback. The nails must not be shorter than the flesh around it. If the nails are short, pressure from the shoes may direct the nail to grow into the tissue. fig
- Shoes should fit properly. Shoes that place too much pressure on the toes or pinch them may cause a nail to grow into the surrounding tissue.

When to seek medical advice:

- Severe pain and discomfort in the toes.
- Pus formation around the toenail.
- Corners of the toenail grows within the soft tissue.
- Ingrown toenail with uncontrolled diabetes.

It is best to seek medical advice as soon as ingrown toenail is suspected.

Home care and prevention of chronic foot pain:

- A warm foot bath will relieve the chronic pain of arthritis.
- Cold compression following a minor foot trauma.
- OTC pain relievers: acetaminophen, naproxen etc.
- Topical pain relieving medications.
- Foot massage is beneficial as it improves circulation. A foot roller may be used for massage.
- Wearing well-fitted, well-cushioned and comfortable footwear.
- Use of arch support may help to keep the foot in a stable shape, providing pain relief.
- Changing shoes and types of footwear. The wrong style of shoe, old shoes, or an incorrect shoe size may injure the foot and result in foot pain
- High heeled and narrow toed shoes should be avoided.

- Maintain good foot hygiene practice.
- Never to walk barefooted.
- Maintain a healthy body weight.
- Keep diabetes strictly controlled.
- Stretching exercises should be done before starting sports in the field.
- Night splints for the foot may be used, physician advice is required.

How to maintain good foot hygiene:

- Feet should be kept as clean as the face.
- A gentle soap may be used to clean the feet, paying special attention to clean the space between the toes.
- Feet must be dried well before donning socks. Moisture-wicking socks may be used, and socks should be kept clean and dry.
- Foot powder or anti-fungal powder may be used.
- A good quality moisturizer may be applied before going to bed.
- Nails should be trimmed regularly but must not be cut too short and must not cut-back to prevent ingrown toe nails.

When to seek medical advice:

- Pain following trauma to the foot.
- Pain that is not relieved by home remedies.
- If pain is accompanied by fever, redness, and/or tenderness in the area.
- Unable to walk normally.
- Pain persists for more than a week and disturbs sleep
- Severe pain and swelling in the foot.

Frozen Shoulder

(Adhesive Capsulitis)

'Frozen shoulder' is also called as *adhesive capsulitis*. It is caused by scar tissue that forms in the shoulder joint capsule. Scar tissue makes the shoulder joint capsule thicker, tighter, and less mobile. It causes pain and stiffness in the shoulder. Over time, the shoulder becomes very hard to move.

The shoulder joint is a ball and socket joint between the shoulder blade (scapula), the lateral part of the collar bone (clavicle) and the arm bone (humerus). The scapula is a large, flat, triangular bone that forms the back part of the shoulder. The shoulder joint is formed by the ball (head) of the arm bone (humerus) with the socket (glenoid cavity) of the scapula. The shoulder joint has a wide range of mobility. It is inherently a very unstable joint.

The shoulder joint capsule is lax and permits greater mobility. A thin membrane called the synovial membrane lines the inner surface of the joint capsule. The synovial membrane produces synovial fluid to lubricate the friction surfaces of the joint.

The joint has several bursae. A bursa is a fluid filled sac and acts as a cushion between tendons and other joint structures for easy joint movements.

Adhesive capsulitis, or frozen shoulder, is a condition where the capsule of the joint becomes thick, scarred, and tight, and synovial fluid secretion is reduced. As a result, the joint becomes stiff and movement of the joint causes pain. Symptoms develop gradually, get worse and then eventually go away. This cycle of changes occur over a period of one to three years.

The name 'adhesive capsulitis', comes from the presence of scar tissue adhesions that form between the joint capsule and the head of the arm bone (humerus).

BODY PAIN AND PAIN RELIEF

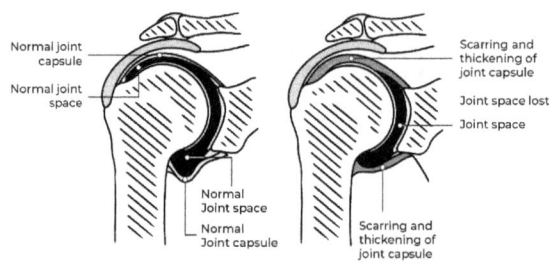

Normal shoulder joint   Frozen shoulder joint

Causes of frozen shoulder:

The exact cause of frozen shoulder is not known.

Risk factors for frozen shoulder:

- Women are more affected than men.
- Between 40 and 60 years of age.
- Diabetes mellitus.
- Shoulder has been immobilized for a longtime due to injury, surgery, or illness.
- Surgery in the shoulder joint and/or breast area.
- Trauma and fracture in the upper limb bones that are then kept immobilized for a prolonged period.
- After a stroke when the arm is not moved for a long time.

Features of frozen shoulder:

- Shoulder joint *stiffness* which makes it difficult or impossible to move the joint.
- Loss of normal range of motion of the shoulder.
- Dull or achy pain in the shoulder region.
- Pain may get worse at night and cause sleep disturbance.
- Difficulty in performing personal activities of daily living.
- The condition worsens with time.

- Quality of life is reduced.
- Range of motion of the joint may go back to normal after 6 months to 2 years.

Home remedies for frozen shoulder:

- OTC pain relievers: ibuprofen, naproxen, acetaminophen.
- The affected joint should be gently moved within the limits of pain and range of movement, which is gradually increased against pain.
- Massage of the affected joint to help relieve tension and tightness and relax the surrounding muscles. Massage can help to restore mobility and improve function by improving blood flow to the affected area and reducing inflammation.
- Warm and cold compress. chart
- Be aware of proper posture:
- Sleep with two pillows, one for the head and the other placed between the elbow and body on the affected side, so that the arm is held slightly away from the body.
- Sleep on the opposite side of the affected shoulder.
- Topical analgesic ointments may be used.

Diet: Anti-inflammatory foods. chart.

Prevention of frozen shoulder:

- The shoulder joint should be kept *mobile*. Prolonged rest to the shoulder joint for any cause can result in *frozen shoulder*.
- Frozen shoulder *exercises*. During exercises, stretching should be done to the point of tension but not pain.

The following exercises are beneficial in preventing the development of frozen shoulder:

- o Pendulum stretch.
- o Towel stretch.
- o Finger walk on the wall.
- o Cross-body reach.
- o Outward rotation.
- o Inward rotation.
- o Arm pit stretch.

BODY PAIN AND PAIN RELIEF

The above exercises should be done under the supervision of a physiotherapist. As the range of motion of the shoulder improves, strengthening exercises of the *'rotator cuff'* may be started under supervision.

- Massage in the shoulder area. benefits:chart.

When to seek medical advice:

- Pain is present even at rest.
- Stiffness of joint gradually increases.
- The intensity of pain changes from an ache to a sharp pain.
- Pain returns when activities are resumed.
- Pain is not subsiding, despite resting the shoulder and refraining from the activities that caused the pain.
- Stiffness of shoulder joint gradually increases.
- Range of movement of the joint gradually decreases.
- Home remedies does not relieve symptoms.

Headache

Every head has its own headache

—ARAB PROVERB

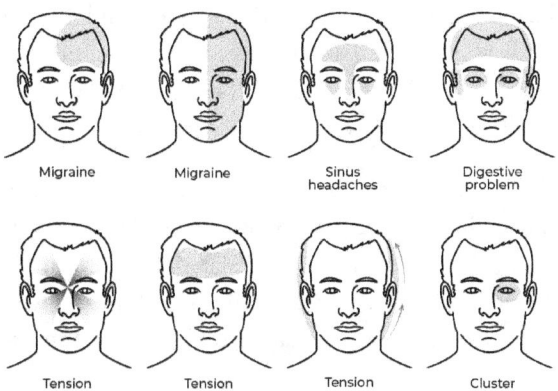

Types of headaches

A Headache is the symptom of pain in the face, head, or neck. The pain felt during a headache comes from a mix of signals between brain, blood vessels, and nearby nerves.

About half of adults have a headache in a given year. Headaches can occur as a result of many conditions, the most common of which is tension headaches, followed by migraine headaches.

According to International Headache Society, the *causes* of headache may include the following conditions:

- Dehydration. Common colds. Sinus problems.
- Fatigue. Stress. Loud noises.
- Sleep deprivation.
- Effects of medicines. Effects of recreational drugs.
- Viral infections. Dental pains.
- Head injury.
- Rapid ingestion of a very cold food or beverages.

The brain has no pain receptors and so the brain itself is not sensitive to pain. However, several areas of the head and neck have *pain receptors* and can thus sense pain. These include the extracranial arteries, middle meningeal artery, large veins, venous sinuses, cranial and spinal nerves, head and neck muscles, the covering of brain (meninges), parts of brain stem, the eyes, the ears, and the teeth which can all be responsible for pain production.

Headaches often result from friction to or irritation of the coverings of brain and blood vessels. The pain receptors may be stimulated by head trauma or tumors, causing headaches. Blood vessel spasms, dilated blood vessels, inflammation, or infection of brain coverings and muscular tension can also stimulate pain receptors. It is very difficult to understand fully the cause of most headaches.

Features of headache:

The characteristics of a headache and the effects on daily life can vary. Some features include:

- Pain affecting one or both sides of the head.
- Pain radiating from a central point.
- Pain is sharp, throbbing, or dull.
- Pain has a vice-like quality, that is a tightening band-like sensation around the head.
- Pain that comes on gradually or suddenly.
- Pain that lasts from under an hour to several days.

The features of pain depend to some extent on the type of headache.

Types of headaches.

There are more than 300 types of headaches, however only about 10% of headaches have a known cause and are called as secondary headaches. The remaining 90% headache types are primary headaches with no known definitive cause.

Primary headache

About 90% of headaches are primary headaches with no known definitive cause. A primary headache is caused by a dysfunction or overactivity of *pain-sensitive* structures in the head.

The structures include:

- The covering of the skull bones.
- Skin and associated soft tissues.
- Muscles of head and neck.
- Eyes. Ears.Teeth.
- Arteries and veins.
- Lining tissues of sinuses, nose, and throat.

Primary headache does not involve an underlying disease in these structures. Instead, chemical activities in the brain, nerves, or blood vessels of the head outside the skull and combination of all these factors may play a role in primary headaches. Primary headaches may also be due to some *genes* and may run in families.

The most common *primary headaches* are:

- Tension headache.
- Migraine.
- Cluster headache.
- Trigeminal headache.

Lifestyle factors that contribute to primary headaches:

- Lack of sleep. Changes in sleep pattern.
- Poor posture.
- Skipped meals.
- Certain foods. Foods containing nitrates. Alcohol.

BODY PAIN AND PAIN RELIEF

Tension headaches

Tension headaches are the most common type of headache among adults and teens. Tension headaches cause mild to moderate pain and come and go over time, typically with no other symptoms.

Features of *tension* headache:

- Headache lasting from 30 minutes to 7 days.
- Non-pulsating pain of mild to moderate intensity.
- Pressing or tightening pain encircling the head like a band, sometimes coming from the neck.
- No aggravation of headache due to walking stairs or similar routine activities.
- Typically *do not* disturb sleep.
- Most people can work through a tension headache.

Home remedies for tension headache:

- Proper hydration maintained by drinking plenty of water.
- Application of hot or cold pack to the head.
- Long hot shower.
- OTC pain relievers: acetaminophen, naproxen, ibuprofen.
- Taking rest in a dark room. Adequate sleep.
- Tea or coffee.
- Reducing chewing activities.
- Supplementation of vitamin B-complex, and magnesium.
- Avoid histamine containing foods: chart
- Maintaining a good posture:

    Standing: shoulder and head should be in the same plane.

    Sitting: thighs should be parallel to the ground and head and trunk should be in the same plane.

- Yoga and mind relaxation.
- Essential oils applied to the forehead or temples.

When to seek medical advice for tension headaches:

- Long-standing tension-type headache.
- Sudden severe headache.
- Headache associated with fever, weight loss, vomiting and/or seizure.

Migraine headaches

Migraine headaches are intense throbbing and pounding pain that can last from 4 hours to 3 days, and usually occur one to four times a month. Migraine headaches are usually associated with sensitivity to light, noise or smells, nausea or vomiting, loss of appetite and upset stomach or belly pain.

Typical features:

- Intense pain in and around eyes.
- Unilateral location.
- Nausea and vomiting. Vision change.
- Speech problems, slurred speech.
- Tingling and numbness in the hands and feet.
- Moderate or severe pain that inhibits daily activities.
- Triggered by stress, hormone fluctuation, sleep disturbances, loud sounds, bright light, strong smell etc.
- Aggravated by climbing stairs or similar routine physical activities.

Home remedies for *migraine headache*:

- Cool the head region by placing an ice pack to the forehead, scalp, and neck region.
- OTC pain relievers: ibuprofen, naproxen, piroxicum.
- A dark, quiet room is very helpful. Sufficient sleep.
- Never to skip a meal. Eating at about the same time everyday.
- Self-relaxation and enjoyment.
- Regular physical exercises. Yoga and meditation.

Avoid some foods:

- Processed foods. Processed meat.
- Bakery foods containing MSG (flavour enhancer).
- Artificial sweeteners. Excess red meat. Yeast.
- Alcohol, red wine, coffee, Caffeinated beverages.
- Dairy products, chocolate, eggs.
- Citrus fruits, tomatoes, onions.

Good foods for migraines:

- Whole rice. Brown rice. Brown bread.
- Lean meat, fish.
- Plain water.

- Orange, yellow, and green colored vegetables.
- Sweet potatoes. Non-citrus fruits. Bananas. Berries.

Cluster headaches

Cluster headaches are the *most severe* type of headache. Cluster headaches are a neurological disorder characterized by recurrent severe headache on *one side* of the head, typically around the eye. During a cluster headache, the patient experiences intense burning or piercing pain behind or around one eye. The pain can be throbbing or constant. The patient cannot sit still and will often walk at a steady and consistent speed especially back and forth during an attack.

Risk factors and causes of cluster headache:

- The exact cause is unknown.
- Males are more affected.
- Family history of cluster headaches.
- Abnormalities in the hypothalamus. Hypothalamus is the body's biological clock situated in the brain.
- Cluster headaches are not associated with triggers such as foods, hormones, or stress.
- Nitroglycerine, a drug used to treat heart disease, smoking and alcohol may trigger the condition.

Typical features of cluster headaches:

- Begins between ages 20 and 45.
- Men are more affected than women.
- Severe or very severe pain.
- Short duration, averaging 45 to 60 minutes.
- Clustering of attacks, generally one to ten episodes of attack in a day.
- Pain starts at the same time each day or the same time every year with no headache between the cluster cycles.
- Pain is unilateral in the orbital, supraorbital and temporal area, with *congestion* of the eye.
- Headache is accompanied by ipsilateral tearing of the eye, nasal congestion, and/or runny nose, eyelid swelling, forehead or facial sweating, constricted pupil and drooping of eyelid.
- Patient is extremely restless and agitated.

Home remedies for cluster headache:

Always *talk to physician* first before starting any home remedies.
- Deep breathing exercises to increase oxygen in the brain.
- Following a consistent sleep schedule.
- Regular physical activities: benefits:chart
- Yoga and meditation.
- OTC pain relievers can help in the initial period.
- OTC topical capsaicin cream.
- Psilocybin mushrooms.
- Ginger tea.
- Use of peppermint essential oil for the scalp.
- Supplementation of magnesium, Vitamin B_2 (riboflavin).
- Avoid alcohol and smoking.

When to seek medical advice:
- If cluster headache was previously diagnosed, the pain alone indicates to seek medical advice.
- Sudden severe headache.

Sinus headaches

Sinuses are air spaces in the nasal passages that help with air humidification and mucus secretion. Inflammation of the sinuses may decrease the ability for the mucus to drain due to increased mucus thickness, causing the passageways of the sinuses to become blocked. This results in increased pressure within the sinuses and can cause a sinus headache.

With sinus headaches, patients will feel a deep and constant pain in the cheek bones, forehead, or on the bridge of nose. Since sinus headaches occurs when the cavities or sinuses in the head become inflamed, the pain usually occurs with other sinus symptoms, like a runny nose, fullness in the ears, fever, and a swollen face. A true sinus headache results from a sinus infection, so the viscus material that comes out of the nose will be yellow or green, unlike the clear discharge in cluster or migraine headache.

Home remedies for sinus headaches:
- Warm compress to the face, nose, and forehead.
- Steam inhalation. Long steam shower.

- Proper hydration of the body by drinking lots of warm plain water to decrease mucus thickness.
- Use of a humidifier. OTC pain relievers.
- Yoga can help to drain mucus from sinus passageways.

Foods that are beneficial in sinus headache:

- Colored vegetables: Sweet potatoes, pumpkin.
- Colored fruits: Papaya, pineapples, red grapes.
- Cinnamon, green leafy vegetables, ginger, berries.
- Foods containing quercetin: Green tea, onion, apples.

When to seek medical advice:

- High fever. Severe headache.
- Swelling around the eye.
- Red and inflamed skin in face and nose.

Hypertension headache

Headache is a feature of hypertension.

Features of hypertension headache:

- Pulsating, throbbing, and early *morning* headache.
- Unilateral or bilateral headache.
- Headache typically worsens with *any activity*.
- Headache may be associated with:
    - Nausea and vomiting. Dizziness.
    - Chest pain. Shortness of breath.
    - Changes in vision. Nosebleed.
    - Tingling and numbness in the fingers.

Home remedies for hypertension headache:

- Strict control of blood pressure.
- Maintaining proper hydration.
- Adequate sleep.
- Cold compress applied to the head.
- Alcohol and fermented beverages should be reduced.
- Vitamin B-complex supplementation.
- Magnesium-containing diet: chart.
- Avoid histamine rich foods: chart.

- Use of essential oils: Lemon, Lavender, Peppermint.

When to seek medical advice:

- *Hypertensive crisis,* which is characterized by:
  - Severe headache. Change in vision.
  - Nausea and vomiting. Nosebleed.
  - Severe anxiety. Seizures.
  - Chest pain. Shortness of breath.

Hormonal headache.

Hormonal headache occurs in women due to shifting hormone levels during menstruation, pregnancy, and menopause. Hormone changes from birth control pills and hormone replacement therapy can also trigger headaches.

Home remedies for hormonal headache:

- Proper hydration by drinking plenty of plain water.
- Cold compression applied to the head.
- Avoid skipping breakfast or any meal.
- Blood sugar levels should be maintained in optimum level by avoiding fasting and eating frequent small snacks. Eating a small snack before going to bed can be beneficial.
- Practice a regular sleep pattern, avoiding too much or too little sleep.
- Self-care, avoiding stress. OTC pain relievers.
- Regular physical exercise to relax the body and mind.
- Supplementation of Magnesium, Riboflavin, and vitamin B-complex. Turmeric and ginger can also help.
- Relaxation exercises: deep breathing, yoga, meditation.

Rebound headache.

Rebound headaches are also known as medication overuse headaches. If pain reliever drugs are used for prolonged period, for instance for more than two or three times a week, or more than 10 days in a month, this type of headache can occur. The same medications that initially relieve headache pain can themselves trigger subsequent headaches if they are used too often. When the pain reliever wears off, the headache comes back and to stop the headache more drug is required. This can cause a dull, constant tension type headache and often it worsens in the morning. The pain may occur daily.

BODY PAIN AND PAIN RELIEF

A person with a history of tension headaches or migraines can suffer from rebound headaches.

Features of rebound headache:

- Dull and constant headache.
- Light and sound sensitivity. Irritability. Restlessness.
- Insomnia. Nausea and vomiting. Constipation.

Home remedies and prevention:

- Headache medications should be taken in limited doses.
- Pain relievers should only be taken when it is truly needed.
- Consultation must be sought for taking pain medications.
- Coffee, if taken before pain starts can be beneficial.
- OTC pain relievers: acetaminophen and aspirin.
- Sedative for sleep.
- Regular physical exercises. chart
- Consultation with a psychotherapist.

Exercise-induced headache

During exercise, the muscles in the head, neck and scalp need more blood supply. The blood vessels swell to increase their supply. Due to a sudden stretching of the blood vessels, pain begins. This type of headache is also called a primary exertional headache and is harmless.

Exertional headaches are a pulsating type of pain on both sides of head lasting between 5 minutes to 48 hours. This type of pain typically occurs during exercise or just afterwards. Exercises that can induce these types of headaches include running, swimming, sexual intercourse, and weightlifting.

Sometimes serious problems are associated with exercise induced headache including brain tumor, bleeding of the brain, or a tumor outside the brain. These are called secondary exercise headaches.

Features of primary exercise headaches:

- Exact cause is unknown.
- Headache is throbbing or pulsating.
- Occurs during or after strenuous exercise.
- Affects both sides of the head in most cases.

Features of secondary exercise headaches:

- Occurs due to underlying causes.
- Same features of primary exercise headaches.
- Vomiting. Rigid neck.
- Vision defects. Congestion in the face and/or eye.
- Loss of consciousness.

Home remedies and prevention:

- Slowly and proper warm-up of the body before starting exercise. Never start exercise while fasted.
- Drinking plenty of water and proper hydration before starting exercise. Drinking sports drinks is beneficial.
- Reducing exercise intensity.

When to seek medical advice:

- Home remedies do not relieve pain.
- Features of *secondary exercise* induced headache are present.

Fasting headaches

Low blood sugar levels have been linked to fasting headaches. However, the exact cause of fasting headaches is not clearly known. In some cases, a genetic correlation has been found. Genetically predisposed people may suffer from headache due to small changes in the blood glucose levels. Blood glucose changes may also alter pain sensation in the brain and cause a fasting headache. Migraine attacks are specially associated with fasting.

Features of fasting headache:

- Low blood sugar may be a feature.
- This is like tension-type headache.
- Pain is typically mild to moderate in intensity.
- Pain is diffuse, in the forehead, and is non-throbbing.
- Pain occurs after at least 16 hours of fasting and resolves within 72 hours after resumption of food intake.
- People who have an underlying headache disorder may be more vulnerable to a fasting-related headache.

Home remedies and prevention:

- Never to skip a meal.
- Eat adequate meals around the same time each day.
- In circumstances when prolonged fasting is expected, a bite of sugar cube, sweet biscuits or even a little food may be taken to prevent the onset of headache. Sports drinks are also helpful.
- Drink plenty of water.
- Cold compress applied to the head.
- Adequate sound sleep.
- Magnesium and vitamin B-complex supplementation.

When to seek medical advice:

- If home remedies do not relieve pain, medical advice should be sought.

Post-traumatic headache

Post-traumatic stress headaches typically start 2-3 days after a head injury and may last for a few months. Typical features include:

- A dull ache that gets worse from time to time.
- Vertigo. Lightheadedness.
- Trouble in concentrating. Problems with memory.
- Tiring quickly. Irritability.

Spinal headache

This type of headache occurs after a spinal tap, a spinal block, or an epidural and is caused due to injury to the spinal coverings. If spinal fluid leaks through the puncture site, it can also cause headache.

Thunderclap headache

Thunderclap headaches are the worst type of headache as they come on suddenly out of nowhere and peak quickly. Thunderclap headaches strike suddenly like a clap of thunder and are an uncommon type of headache. Thunderclap headache may be a warning of a potentially life-threatening condition. Urgent medical attention is necessary.

Causes of thunderclap headache:

- Head injury. Brain blood vessel tear, rupture, or blockage.
- Stroke from a ruptured blood vessel in the brain.
- Ischemic stroke from a blocked blood vessel in the brain.

- Narrowed and inflamed blood vessels in the brain.
- Blood pressure changes in late pregnancy.

Any sudden or new headache should be taken very seriously as it is often the only warning sign of a serious problem.

Features of *thunderclap* headache:

- Sudden and severe pain in the head.
- Pain reaches its most intense point within 60 seconds and lasts at least 5 minutes.
- Numbness and weakness in the limbs.
- Speech problems, slurred speech.
- Nausea and vomiting. Vision changes.
- Confusion and change of mental state.
- Seizures. Change in sensation.
- Fever.

When to seek medical advice:

Immediate medical advice must be sought.

Headache due to dehydration

When the body is dehydrated, the brain can temporarily shrink from fluid loss. This mechanism causes the brain to pull away from the skull, causing pain. This phenomenon is called a dehydration headache. Once rehydrated, the brain returns to normal state and thus relieves the headache.

Causes of dehydration:

- Not drinking enough water or fluids.
- Losing more fluid than fluid taken.
- Increased loss of fluid through diarrhea, vomiting, urination or sweat.

Features of dehydration headache:

- Dull headache. Pain in all sides of the head.
- No pain in the face.
- Sometimes intense migraine-like headache.

Home remedies for dehydration headache:

- Increased fluid intake.
- Consuming electrolyte drinks: Coconut water, fruit juices, sports drinks, milk.
- Temporarily reduce all physical activities.
- Avoid heat to reduce sweating.

Headache due to brain tumor

Headache due to a brain tumor may be severe and worsen with activity or occur in the early morning. It may also be accompanied by different types of seizures, personality or memory changes, nausea or vomiting, fatigue, drowsiness, and problems with sleep.

Any case of suspected brain tumor should be consulted immediately with a physician.

Headache due to eye problems

Prolonged and hard working of the eyes will cause the eyes to strain much. The eye muscles may contract too much. These contractions can cause a strain headache. There are many other eye problems which may cause headache.

Common causes are:

- Prolonged straining of eye.
- Increased pressure within the eye (glaucoma).
- Vision defects. Lens defects (cataract).

Features of eye problems:

- Sore and tired eyes.
- Watery or dry eyes.
- Increased sensitivity to light.
- Burning or itching eyes.
- Neck pain. Shoulder or back pain.
- Vision problems. Difficulty in keeping eyes open.
- Difficult to concentrate.

Home remedies and preventions:

- Sufficient sleep.
- Wear of sunglass when outside.

- At every 20 minutes, eyes should be taken off the TV or computer screen to focus for 20 seconds on an object in the distance.
- Massage to the head.
- Hot/cold applications.
- Breathing exercises.
- Proper hydration by drinking fluids. Green tea.
- Avoid some foods: caffeine-containing foods and beverages, MSG containing foods, nitrate containing foods like meats, hotdogs, sausage, pizza etc.

When to see a physician:

- Home remedies donot relieve the headache.
- To find out the cause.
- To correct the vision defects.

Home remedies in the begining for headaches:

- Application of heat or ice pack against the head or neck. Extreme temperatures should be avoided.
- Taking of regular meals and care should be taken to maintain stable blood sugar levels.
- Stress must be avoided whenever possible and use of healthy coping strategies for unavoidable stress.
- Adequate sleep is a must. A regular routine for sleeping must be followed and the bedroom should be calm, quiet, cool, and dark.
- Regular physical exercises to boost overall health and lower stress.
- Drinking plenty of water.
- Taking breaks when working and stretching of body muscles multiple times a day.
- Eye strain must be prevented. Adequate light intensity is essential in the workplace.

Headaches which require prompt medical care:

- Headaches that first develop after the age of 50.
- A major change in the pattern of headaches.
- A severe and sudden headache and gets steadily worse.
- Head pain that increases with coughing or change in posture.
- Headaches accompanied by changes in personality.
- Headache associated with nausea, vomiting and fainting.

- Headaches with fever, stiff neck, confusion, decreased alertness or memory, neurological symptoms such as visual disturbances, slurred speech, weakness, numbness or seizures.
- Headaches with a painful red eye and watering from the eye.
- Headaches accompanied by pain and tenderness in the temples.
- Headaches after a blow and/or trauma to the head.
- Headaches that disturb activities of daily life and/or sleep.
- Headaches with chronic diseases, cancer or impaired immunity.
- Sudden numbness, weakness or paralysis on one side of the body.

Hip Joint Pain

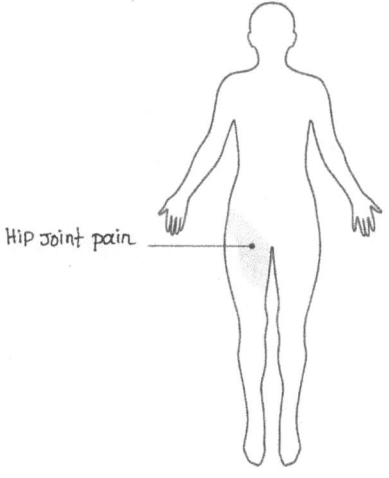

The *'Hip'* and *'Buttock'* are the same place in the body. The hip area is located between the upper part of the thigh and lower part of waist. It is the laterally projecting region of each side of the lower or posterior part of the trunk formed by the lateral parts of the pelvis and upper part of the thigh bone together. Heavy fleshes and fat cover the part.

The groin is the junctional area between the lowest part of the abdomen and the upper thigh on either side of the midline.

The joint at the upper part of the thigh bone is the hip joint and is located in the hip area.

The hip joint is a type of synovial joint known as a ball and socket joint. The ball is the head of the thigh bone and socket is in the hip bone. The inner lining of the joint capsule is covered by a thin membrane called the synovial membrane.

Hip joint forms a connection between the lower limb and the pelvic girdle and thus is designed for stability and weight bearing in both static (standing) and dynamic (walking or running) postures.

The ball shaped head of the thigh bone and the socket of the hip bone are covered by a pain insensitive tissue called cartilage. As such, friction between the ball and socket is painless and we can move and stand normally without pain. However, if this cartilage covering is lost for any reason, the underlying bone, which is very pain sensitive, is exposed and severe pain will be felt in the hip area.

Causes of hip joint pain:
- *Excess body weight* causing increased friction between the bones and eventually erosion of the cartilage covering and pain.
- *Injury* to the hip joint causing sprain or dislocation of joint.
- *Inflammation* of the hip joint: rheumatoid arthritis and osteoarthritis. Pain is felt in the groin and frontal aspect of the thigh.
- *Infection* in the hip joint (septic arthritis) and bones (osteomyelitis).
- *Inflammation* of the synovial membrane.
- Any *fracture* or *dislocation* of bones of the hip joint.
- Strenuous exercises, including excess and unaccustomed running, dancing, and sports activities.
- Sudden change in exercise activities.
- Inflammation of the tendons, ligaments and bursas associated with the hip joint.
- Any *nerve compression* around the hip.
- *Tumors* of the bones of the hip joint.
- Low back pain can sometimes mimic hip pain.
- Reduced blood supply causing necrosis (death) to the head of the thigh bone.
- *Osteoporosis* (porous bone) of the bones of the hip joint.

Features of inflammation *(arthritis)* in the hip joint:
- Pain in the hip joint which is usually felt in the groin region.
- Pain is felt deep into the joint.
- Sometimes pain is felt in the outer part of the hip joint and in the buttocks.
- Pain may extend to front side of the thigh and knee area.
- Pain typically becomes worse in the morning and after a prolonged rest.

- Pain is relieved to some extent with activity.
- Cold weather may increase pain.
- In the later stages, pain is constant and night pain occurs.
- Limping while walking.
- Swelling in the groin area.
- Feeling of stiffness in the joint. A common problem of stiffness in the hip joint is difficulty in putting on shoes or socks.
- Reduced range of motion of the hip joint. Decreased range of motion leads to joint contractures and muscle atrophy leading to weakness in movements of the hip.
- Difficulty in standing-up straight or squatting.
- Pain while trying to put weight on leg on the affected side.
- Fever.
- Pressing in the groin area elicits pain.
- Cracking sound in the hip joint with movement.
- Activities of daily life gradually impaired.
- Apparent limb length discrepancy may be present.
- Deformity of the joint may be seen.

Home remedies for hip pain:

- Hip pain which occurs due to excess and unaccustomed running, dancing, sports activities, and strenuous exercises can be relieved by:
    - Taking rest.
    - Application of cold packs to the groin area.
    - OTC pain relievers: Ibuprofen, Naproxen, piroxicum.
- Direct pressure on the hip should be avoided, such as: bending, sitting, or lying on that side.
- Reduce weight bearing on the affected side while walking by using crutches or a walking stick.
- Gentle muscle stretching and resistance exercises.
- Low impact exercises: walking, swimming, cycling.
- Warm pool swimming.

Prevention of arthritic hip pain:

- Maintaining a healthy body weight.
- Low impact exercises: walking, swimming, and cycling done.
- High impact activities: running, jumping, dancing avoided.
- Avoid activities which initiate pain.
- Wearing proper attire and shoes for sports activities.
- Eating healthy and balanced diet. chart
- Proper warm-up is mandatory before any sports activity.
- Calcium and vitamin D supplementation.
- Stretching exercises for the hip, back, and pelvic muscles.

When to seek medical advice:

- Pain is not relieved after 2 weeks of home treatment.
- Pain accompanied by fever and swelling of the joint.
- Pain just after a trauma or fall to the ground.
- Pain hampers normal activities of daily life.
- Pain in the hip and loss of appetite and body weight.
- Numbness and weakness in the foot.
- Movement of the limb in any direction causes pain.

Septic arthritis of hip joint

Infection of hip joint is *septic arthritis*. Generally single hip joint is affected. It is a serious medical condition and requires immediate and aggressive treatment to prevent permanent damage to the joint.

Features of *septic arthritis* of hip joint:

- Fever, chills and nausea.
- Hip Joint pain. Swelling in the front area of the hip.
- Warm to touch in the groin area.
- Color change in the skin over the groin area.
- Movements of the joint will be lost or reduced and will elicit severe pain.
- Generally, single joint is affected.

Emergency treatment is a must to stop the risks of *permanent* joint damage.

See *joint infection and pain (septic arthritis)*: page:

Joint Infection and Pain

(Septic Arthritis)

Joint infection is called septic arthritis. Septic arthritis is a painful condition. Any joint in the body may be affected. Large joints are commonly affected.

Bacteria and other germs travel through the blood stream from a distant site in the body to the joint and establishes infection. Skin and blood infections, infected wounds in the body or genital infections may act as a source of organisms. Children and older age group people are mainly affected by blood borne infections. Organisms may also reach the joint by a direct injury to the joint, like a penetrating injury to the joint.

Infections destroy the joint surfaces and produce symptoms.

Risk factors for septic arthritis:
- Children, older and debilitated people are more affected.
- Pre-existing joint diseases, like rheumatoid arthritis and osteoarthritis will increase the occurance.
- Poorly controlled or uncontrolled diabetes mellitus.
- Immunosuppressive drugs use and abuse.
- Chronic kidney and liver failure, chronic lung diseases.
- After joint replacement surgery. Septic arthritis causes loosening of the joint.
- Intravenous drug use and abuse.

Which joints are more affected?
- Any joint in the body may be affected. Most often only one joint is affected.
- Large joints are commonly affected: knee, hip, ankle, shoulder, elbow,wrist and joints of the spine.
- Small joints of fingers and toes may also be affected.

Features of infected (septic) arthritis:

- *Severe pain* in the affected joint, especially with movements of the limb.
- Fever and chills.
- Skin over the joint may become red and warm to touch.
- Fatigue and generalized weakness.
- Swelling of the joint due to increased fluid and pus within the joint.
- Sometimes there is inability to move the limb with the infected joint.

When to seek medical advice:

As soon as septic arthritis is suspected, it is better to seek medical advice.

Kidney and Renal Pain

(Renal Colic or Pain)

Renal colic or pain means pain that occurs due to stone or obstruction in the urinary tract. Urinary tract includes the *kidneys, ureters, urinary bladder* and *urethra*.

Kidneys

The kidneys are reddish-brown and bean-shaped organs. They are two in number and are attached with the posterior wall of the abdomen on both right and left sides just with and below the ribs.

Main functions of kidneys are:
- Regulation of body fluid levels.
- Excretion of wastes and toxins.
- Regulation of p^H of body fluids.
- Production of some hormones.

Ureter

a tube that conveys urine from kidney to the Urinary bladder.

Causes of renal stone formation:

Exact cause is not known. There are some risk factors.

Risk factors for renal stone formation:
- *Long standing water deprivation* in the body due to less water intake or increased water loss in warm and dry climates and who sweat a lot will cause accumulation of more crystal-forming substances in the urine and stone formation.
- *Family history* of kidney stone formation.

BODY PAIN AND PAIN RELIEF

- *Dietary* habit is important. Diets high in protein, sodium salt and sugar are at increased risk.
- Chronic diarrhea.
- Inflammatory bowel diseases. Stomach diseases.
- Some metabolic diseases. Obesity.
- Repeated urinary tract infection.
- *Excess vitamin C* supplimentation.
- *Over use* of laxatives, Calcium-based antacids.
- *Congenital abnormality* in the urinary system.
- Any type of obstruction in the kidney and ureter.
- Stone-forming *foods*: Beets, spinach, chocolates, nuts etc.

Features of stone in the kidney:

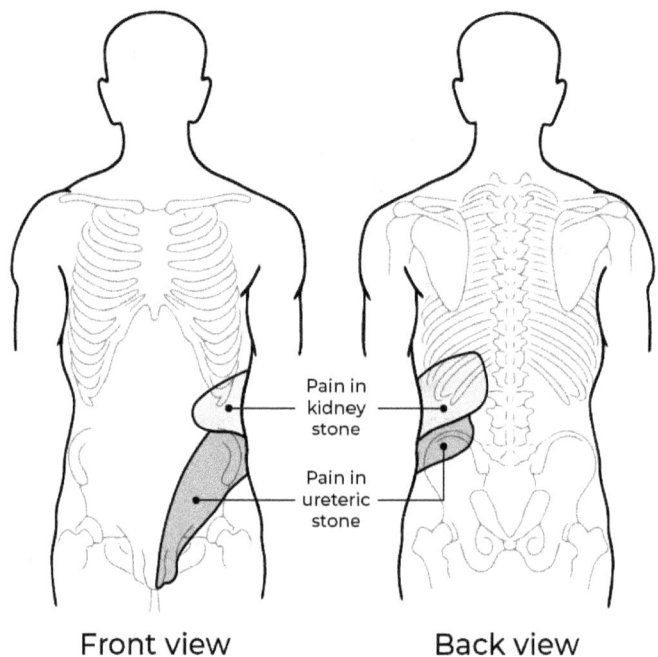

Fig:Sites of renal pain.

- Severe, sharp pain in the side and lower back below the level of ribs and in the loin. This pain is one of the most severe type of pain.

Loin is the part of the body that is situated on each side of the spinal column between the hip bones and the lowest ribs.

- Pain comes in waves and fluctuates in intensity.
- Urine may be cloudy in appearance.
- Pain or burning sensation while urinating.
- Nausea and vomiting.
- Sometimes fever and chills.

Features of stone in the *ureter*:

- Sudden, severe loin pain.
- Pain may radiate to the groin, testis or labia majora.
- Urgent desire to pass urine.
- Increased frequency of micturation.
- Passage of small amount of urine at a time.
- Blood may pass with the urine.

Prevention of renal stone formation:

- Remain physically active. Sedentary lifestyle promotes kidney stone formation. Prolonged bed rest should be avoided.
- Body should be kept hydrated by drinking plenty of water.
- Dietary calcium intake is preferred. Extra calcium supplements intake should be discouraged.
- Limit food with high oxalate content, e.g,
    o All berries especially cranberries.
    o Beets. Spinach. Beans. Sweet potatoes.
    o Peanuts. Coffee, chocolate, Beer.
- Avoid:
    o High salt containing foods.
    o Excess vitamin C suppliments.
    o Excess animal protein.
    o Extra calcium supplements.

Urinary bladder

Urinary bladder is a hollow, distensible muscular organ. It sits on the pelvic floor. Urinary bladder stores urine from the kidneys. Ureters convay urine from the kidneys to the urinary bladder. This urine is disposed via the urethra by urination.

Features of *stone* in the urinary bladder:

- Discomfort or pain in the penis or vulva.
- Lower abdominal pain.
- Frequent urination. Pain during urination.
- Sometimes interruption in urine flow (a start-stop flow).
- Blood in urine.
- Cloudy or abnormally dark-colored urine.

Features of *inflammation* and *infection* of urinary bladder (cystitis):

- Inflammation of urinary bladder is mostly due to an infection.
- Lower abdominal or pelvic pain or discomfort.
- Fever and chills.
- A strong, persistent urge to urinate.
- A burning sensation when urinating.
- Passing frequent, small amount of urine.
- Passing cloudy or strong-smelling urine.
- Associated lower back pain.

Home remedies for *cystitis*:

- Always remain hydrated. Wash out the urinary bladder by taking plenty of water.
- Never hold urine for prolonged period. Urinate when the need arises.
- Probiotic, yogart intake is good.
- Vitamin C and cranberry juice supplimentation is beneficial.
- Practice good sexual hygiene.
    - Always pee just before and after sexual intercourse.
    - Wash the genitals, especially the foreskin before and after having sex or intercourse.
    - Always wipe vulva from *front to behind*.
    - Always use separate tissue paper to wipe anus and vulva.
    - Sexual partners should be awared of any current or previous urinary tract infection.

When infection is suspected, always consult with physician.

Home remedies for *healthy kidneys*:

- Maintenance of proper hydration of body by drinking sufficient water and fluids.
- Avoid alcohol and coffee.

- Healthy and balanced diet.
- Maintenance of healthy body weight.
- Enough sleep.
- Not to sit still for prolonged period. Atleast one minute of walking in every hour is beneficial.

Kidney *friendly* foods:

- Refined bread and rice. Probiotic, yogurt.
- Cabbage. Cauliflower.
- Pineapple. Red grapes. Radish. Garlic. Onion. Turnip.
- Olive oil. Egg white. Skinless chicken.
- Vitamin C suppliments.

Foods *bad* for kidney:

- Canned foods. Packaged meals.
- Whole wheat bread. Brown rice.
- Excess sugar. Potatoes and sweet potatoes.
- Processed meats. Too much meat. Alcohol. Soda.
- Dairy products. Chips. Crackers.
- Bananas. Oranges. Spinach. Tomatoes. Dates. Apricots.
- Avocados. Prunes. Raisins. Pickles. Olives. Relish.

When to seek medical advice:

It is better to seek medical advice as early as it is suspected.

Urinary tract infection (UTI)

Urinary system consists of:
- *Kidneys:* form urine.
- *Ureters:* convey urine from kidneys to urinary bladder.
- *Urinary bladder*: stores urine.
- *Urethra:* expels urine from the urinary bladder to the exterior.

Urinary tract infection (UTI) is an infection in any part of the urinary system. Most of the urinary infections involve the lower urinary tract. Lower urinary tract includes the *urinary bladder* and the *urethra*.

Woman urethra is very short (4-5 cm) as compared to male urethra (18-20 cm). Woman urethra is in direct contact with the external genital organs like vulva and vagina. So, women are at a greater risk of developing an UTI than are men.

BODY PAIN AND PAIN RELIEF

Features of UTI:

- Persistent pelvic and lower abdominal pain.
- Fever and chills.
- A strong and persistent urge to urinate.
- Urine leakage.
- A burning sensation during urination.
- A feeling of incomplete urination.
- Lower back pain.
- Passing frequent, small amounts of urine.
- Require to urinate at night.
- Cloudy urine due to mix of blood.
- Strong-smelling urine.
- Feeling of pressure in the lower pelvis.
- Pain during sex.
- Feeling of fatigue.

Home remedies and prevention for UTI:

- Proper hydration of the body by drinking plenty of water.
- Never to delay urination. Never to hold urine for too long. When need arises, must empty the bladder.
- Women should wash or wipe her vulva from front to back. Never from back to front.
- Good and safe sex hygiene should be practiced.
- Always urination should be complete. Bladder should be kept empty.
- Must urinate just after sexual intercourse.
- OTC pain relievers: Acetaminophen, Naproxen, Ibuprofen.
- Use of heat pad can soothe the area.

Good foods in UTI:

- Probiotic yogurt. Whole grains.
- Vegetables. Green beans. Squash. White and sweet potatoes.
- Bananas. Nuts. Garlic.
- Lean protein: poultry. fish. eggs.
- Black and green tea. Dark chocolate.
- Vitamin C supplimentation.

Foods to avoid in UTI:

- Caffeine. Alcohol.
- Spicy foods. Citrus fruits.
- Nicotine. Smoking. Carbonated drinks.
- Artificial sweetners.
- Excess meat.

When to seek medical advice:

It is better to seek medical advice as early as it is suspected.

Sexually transmitted diseases (STD)

Sexually transmitted diseases are infections that are passed from one person to another through sexual contact. The contact is usually vaginal, oral and anal sex. Sometimes they can spread through other intimate physical contact.

Features of STD:

- Sores on the genitals.
- Lower abdominal and pelvic pain.
- Painful micturation.
- Odd-smelling vaginal discharge.
- Discharge from the penis.
- Pain during sex in women.
- Pain in bowel movements and in micturation.
- Pain in testes.

Prevention of STDs:

- Limit sex partners.
- Before having sex, get sexual histories of the partner.
- Before having sex, tests for venereal diseases may be done.
- Sexual contact should be avoided under the influence of alcohol or drug.
- Vaccination against some infections: HBV, HPV.
- Barrier methods (condom) should be used every time before engaging in sexual activity.
- Maintaining good hygiene habits before and after sexual contact:
  - Rinsing off after sexual contact.
  - Urinating after sex to help to prevent UTI.
- Correct use of condoms and other barrier methods.
- Must to observe partners for any:

BODY PAIN AND PAIN RELIEF

- o Sore in the genitalia.
- o Discharges from the genital tract.
- o Any needle tract in the body.

When to seek medical advice:

It is better to seek medical advice as early as it is suspected.

Liver Pain

'Is life worth living? It all depends on the liver'.

—William James

Liver is a reddish-brown wedge-shaped organ. It is the largest organ in the body. Weight is about 1.5kg. Liver is situated just under the rib cage on the right side of abdomen. Liver cells can regenerate.

Functions of liver:

- Helps in digestion of foods.
- Breakdown of nutrients (metabolism).
- Synthesis of nutrients and blood clotting factors.
- Blood detoxification and filtration.
- Storage of sugars, vitamins and minerals.
- Excretion of drugs and chemicals.

Causes of liver pain:

- Infection and inflammation of liver by viruses:
    - Hepatitis A virus (HAV).
    - Hepatitis B virus (HBV).
    - Hepatitis C virus (HCV).
- Alcoholic hepatitis.
- Pus formation in the liver.
- Tumors and cancers in the liver.
- Fatty liver disease.
- Congenital abnormalities in the liver.

Features of liver diseases:

- Abdominal pain or discomfort, especially on the right upper abdomen beneath the lower ribs.
- Swelling in abdomen, legs and ankles.

- Yellow coloration of skin and eyes. Skin itching.
- Loss of appetite. Nausea and vomitting.
- Fatigue and generalized weakness.
- Dark urine and pale stool may be present.

Home remedies for long term liver diseases:

- Maintenence of healthy body weight.
- Physical activities of daily life should be continued.
- Healthy and balanced diet.chart
- Regular physical exercises: walking, swimming.
- Control of diabetes and high blood pressure.
- Control of high blood cholesterol level.
- Refined sugar and fat should be avoided in the diet.
- Yoga and meditition.

Liver *friendly* foods:

- Drinking of plenty of water. Green tea.
- Whole cereals, brown rice, Oatmeal, quinoa, barley.
- Foods containing omega-3 fatty acids. chart
- Fish and sea foods, Lean meats, poultry, egg white.
- Fresh fruits and leafy green vegetables: Berries, avocados, papya, papya seeds, gooseberry, apples, any citrus fruit.
- Garlic, Turmeric, lemon, olive oils, peas, lentils, pulses, legumes. cauliflower, broccoli.
- Yogurt, milk.

Foods *bad* for liver.

- Alcohol. Refined cereals, refined bread, rice.
- Added sugar and sugary foods.
- High fat foods. Added salt in diet.
- Fried foods. French fries. Red meat.
- Saturated fats: Butter. Cream. High-fat dairy foods. Fatty meats.
- Bakery foods, cookies, cake, packaged baked foods.

Hepatitis A (HAV)

It is an infection and inflammation of the liver cells. It is caused by the hepatitis A virus. The viral infection cause inflammation and affect the normal functions of the liver. The disease spreads by the contaminated foods and water.

Features of HAV:

- Feeling of fatigue, weakness and lethargic.
- Sudden nausea and vomiting.
- Yellow coloration of eye (white area of eyeball looks yellow), oral cavity lining and skin.
- Abdominal pain or discomfort, especially on the right upper abdomen beneath the lower ribs.
- Loss of appetite. Low grade fever. Joint pain.

Generally, the features are relatively mild and go away in a few weeks. Sometimes the features of hepatitis A are severe and lasts for several months.

Home remedies for hepatitis A:

- Stay at home. Strictly be in rest in bed.
- Large meals should be avoided.
- Take small and frequent meals. Glucose and carbohydrate drinks are beneficial.
- Remain hydrated. Plenty of water intake.
- Avoid alcohol and smoking.
- Separate yourself from other members of the family.

When to seek medical advice:

- Severe weakness and feeling of fatigue.
- Yellow skin, mouth cavity and eyes.
- Pain and discomfort in the abdomen.
- Nausea and vomiting that does not improve by 1-2 days.

Hepatitis B (HBV)

Hepatitis B is a serious liver infection caused by the hepatitis B virus. Infection may range from mild to severe. The virus spreads from person to person through blood, semen, saliva, vaginal secretion or other body fluids. Sometimes hepatitis B virus infection becomes chronic and lasts more than six months. HBV infection increases the risk of developing cirrhosis of liver, liver cancer and liver failure. In cirrhosis the liver gets permanently scarred. Most adults with hepatitis B infection recover fully, but there is no cure for HBV infection.

BODY PAIN AND PAIN RELIEF

Risk factors for hepatitis B virus infection:

- Use of sharing needles during drug use and abuse.
- Unprotected sex with multiple sex partners with HBV.
- Baby born to an infected mother.
- Men who have sex with men with HBV.

Hepatitis B virus does not spread by:

- Food or water. Sharing eating utensils.
- Breast feeding.
- Hugging. Kissing. Hand holding.
- Coughing. Sneezing.

Features of hepatitis B virus infection:

- General sense of feeling of unwell.
- Right upper abdominal pain.
- General body pains and aches.
- Loss of appetite. Nausea and vomiting.
- Weakness, tiredness, and extreme fatigue.
- Fever. Joint pain.
- Yellow coloration of skin, mouth cavity and white area of eyes.
- Diarrhea. Dark colored urine, clay colored stool.
- Features of liver failure.

Features of liver failure:

- Yellow coloration of skin and eye balls.
- General feeling of sense of unwell.
- Nausea and vomitting.
- Abdominal swelling.
- Pain in right upper abdomen. Tremors.
- Disorientation or confusion. Sleepiness.
- Breath may have a sweet odour.

Home remedies:

- Sufficient bed rest.
- Maintain a cool and well-ventilated environment.
- Healthy and balanced diet.
- Healthy body weight.
- Diabetes and hypertention controlled.

When to seek medical advice:

It is better to seek medical advice as early as it is suspected exposure to hepatitis B virus.

Inflammation of Gallbladder (cholecystitis)

Gallbladder is a small pouch like organ attached to the undersurface of liver. Gallbladder stores bile. Bile is produced by the liver cells. Bile is a digestive fluid and is required for the digestion and absorption of fat and fat-soluble vitamins in food.

A *gallstone* is a stone formed within the gallbladder out of precipitated bile components. Bile components are cholesterol, bile salts, bilirubin and calcium. They combindly form stone-like hard particles.

Causes of inflammation of gallbladder:

- *Stones and infection* in gallbladder.
- Tumor in the gallbladder.
- *Blockage* of gallbladder passage by stone or tumor.

Features of inflammation of gallbladder:

- Sudden and rapidly increasing pain in the upper right or central part of the belly especially after a fatty meal.
- Pain may be felt in the right shoulder.
- Back pain may be felt between the shoulder blades.
- Indigestion. Gas in the stomach. Heartburn.
- Fever and chills.
- Pain is not relieved by taking anti-ulcerant drugs.

Prevention of *gallstone* formation:

- Maintenance of healthy body weight. Obesity is one of the most common cause for gallstone formation.
- Taking of healthy fat: chart
- High fiber and low fat diet.
- Regular physical exercises. Sedentary lifestyle increases the chance of stone formation.
- Avoid: white bread, white pasta, refined cereals, Animal fats and too much fatty food.

BODY PAIN AND PAIN RELIEF

When to seek medical advice:

It is better to seek medical advice as early as it is suspected.

Knee Pain

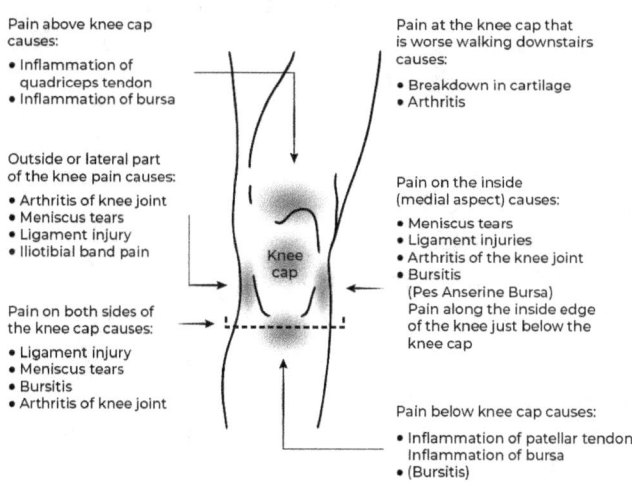

Pain around knee joint

Pain above knee cap causes:
- Inflammation of quadriceps tendon
- Inflammation of bursa

Outside or lateral part of the knee pain causes:
- Arthritis of knee joint
- Meniscus tears
- Ligament injury
- Iliotibial band pain

Pain on both sides of the knee cap causes:
- Ligament injury
- Meniscus tears
- Bursitis
- Arthritis of knee joint

Pain at the knee cap that is worse walking downstairs causes:
- Breakdown in cartilage
- Arthritis

Pain on the inside (medial aspect) causes:
- Meniscus tears
- Ligament injuries
- Arthritis of the knee joint
- Bursitis
  (Pes Anserine Bursa)
  Pain along the inside edge of the knee just below the knee cap

Pain below knee cap causes:
- Inflammation of patellar tendon
  Inflammation of bursa
- (Bursitis)

© Dr. Abu Hena Mahboob

Knee is the largest joint in the body. The knee joins the thigh with the leg. Thigh bone is the femur and leg bone is the tibia. One small flat bone called patella (knee cap) acts as a cap of the knee joint. The ends of bones forming the knee joint is covered by a pain insensitive tissue called cartilage. Due to the presence of pain insensitive cartilage we can move the joint painless. If this cartilage covering is lost by any reason, the underlying bone which is pain sensitive is exposed and severe pain will be felt in the knee area.

The knee joint consists of two joints. One between the thigh bone (femur) and the leg bone (tibia) and the other between the femur and the knee cap (patella).

The knee joint as a whole is covered by a capsule. The inner wall of the capsule is lined by synovial membrane. The synovial membrane secretes a lubricating fluid called synovial fluid. Synovial fluid lubricates the moving surfaces of the joint and we can move the joint comfortably.

Knee is a hinge-type of joint and helps in bending and straightening the leg. It also permits slight rotational movements.

Knee pain is the pain which is experienced in and around the knee joint. Pain may be on the anterior aspect or on the sides. Pain on the posterior aspect of the knee is generally a radiated pain from the lower back region. Knee pain may extend from lower thigh to upper leg.

Causes of knee pain:
- Trauma to the knee. Knee sprain.
- Erosion and inflammation (osteoarthritis) of the knee joint. Osteoarthritis mostly seen in older age group, as age increases the incidence of osteoarthritis also increases. This is the commonest type. Secondary osteoarthritis may occur in younger people.
- Inflammation of the knee joint. Rheumatoid arthritis is a common example. Cause is not known. Middle aged people are mainly affected.
- Infection in knee joint. It is called septic arthritis.
- Tumour in bones around the knee.
- Inflammation and tumor of tissues in and around knee.

Factors predisposing knee pain:
- *Family history* of knee pain.
- *Trauma* to the knee. Knee sprain.
- *Older age:* increases the incidence of pain.
- *Obesity. Diabetes mellitus. Smoking.*
- Hard *physical labour. Stress* and *anxiety.*

Symptoms associated with knee pain:
Symptoms depend on the cause.

Symptoms those accompany knee pain include:
- Swelling of the knee. Stiff knee joint.
- Pain increases with movement of the knee during walking, sitting, standing from sitting position.
- Skin color may be changed.

- Feeling of warmth over the joint. Fever.
- Weakness in the limb.
- Insecured feeling on standing and walking.
- Crunching and popping noise during walking and squat.
- It may be impossible to full straightening and bending the knee.

Knee sprain

Knee sprain is the injury to the knee joint. It is due to torn or overstretching of the ligaments and the tissues which hold the bones together and gives stability to the joint.

Features of *knee sprain:*

- Knee sprain is the commonest knee injury.
- Pain in the knee after a direct blow or twisting injury.
- Popping sound is heard by the patient during injury.
- Swelling of the knee joint. Weakness in the limb.
- Pain on movement and on standing and walking.
- Knee buckling under a weight or on standing.
- Walking with a limp.
- Feeling of *'give out'* with standing and walking.
- Knee stiffness.

When to seek medical advice:

As soon as knee sprain is suspected, immediate medical advice should be taken.

Infection of knee joint (septic arthritis)

Infection of knee joint is *septic arthritis*. Generally single knee joint is affected. It is a serious medical condition and requires immediate and aggressive treatment to prevent permanent damage to the joint.

Features of *septic arthritis* of knee joint:

- Fever, chills and nausea.
- Knee Joint pain. Swelling around the knee.
- Knee feels warm to touch.
- Color change in the skin over the knee joint.
- Movements of the joint will be lost or reduced and will elicit severe pain.
- Generally, single joint is affected.

Emergency treatment is a must to stop the risks of permanent joint damage.

See also septic arthritis page:261.

Osteoarthritis of knee joint

In osteoarthritis, there is erosion and inflammation of tissues associated with the knee joint.

Osteoarthritis is the commonest form of joint disease throughout the world. It is strongly associated with age, and extremely common in older people.

Factors those increase the risk of osteoarthritis. see *osteoarthritis*. page

Features of osteoarthritis in knee:

- *Pain* in the knee during and after movement and even during taking a rest.
- *Pain* on touching and pressing the joint.
- *Swelling* of the knee joint.
- *Stiff* knee. Stiffness mostly present in the morning after awakening and after a period of inactivity.
- *Loss of flexibility*. Range of movement of the joint is reduced.
- *Grating sensation* on bending or straightening of the knee.
- Knee becomes *'knobby'* in appearance.

Prevention of pain in osteoarthritis. see osteoarthritis

Prevention of injury to the knee joint:

- Avoid bending knees past 90^0 when doing half-knee bends.
- Prevent twisting the knees during exercises.
- Do warm-up exercises before sports.
- When jumping, land with knees bent.
- Properly fitted shoes is a must, that provide shock absorption and stability. Shoe inserts may be used.
- Exercise on soft surface.
- Avoid running on asphalt and concrete.

Benefits of exercises for osteoarthritis.

Exercise is considered as the most effective, non-drug treatment for reducing pain and improving movements in patients with osteoarthritis. Exercises should be done under supervision.

Exercises are:
- *Range of motion* or,flexibility exercises: these exercises can help to maintain and improve the flexibility in the joint.
- *Walking:* Benefits:chart.
- *Strengthening exercises:* These exercises help to mainten and improve muscle strength. Strong muscles can support and protect joints that are affected by arthritis.
- *Aquatic (water) exercises:* Beneficial for the overweight. They are performed while standing in about shoulder-height water.

See also osteoarthritis page: 320.

Rheumatoid arthritis (RA)

Rheumatoid arthritis is a systemic disease. It affects whole body organs.

Causes of rheumatoid arthritis. see rheumatoid arthritis

Features of rheumatoid arthritis in knee:
- Pain and swelling in knee joint.
- Joints are painful to touch.
- Stiffness and reduced range of movement of knee.
- Stiffness is marked in the morning and lasts for 1 hour.
- Features present on both knees.
- Loss of appetite and weight loss.
- Generalised weakness and fatigue.
- fever.

See also rheumatoid arthritis page 381.

Foods and knee pain.

Foods to *avoid* in Rheumatoid arthritis and Osteoarthritis.

Foods which cause inflammation: chart

Foods beneficial in Rheumatoid arthritis and Osteoarthritis.They reduce inflammation. chart

BODY PAIN AND PAIN RELIEF

Home remedies for knee pain:

Mild to moderate knee pain can often be treated at home.

Following home remedies may be helpfull:
- Rest to the knee joint. Prolonged rest is not advised. One minute of walking in every hour is beneficial.
- Elevation of the knee to reduce knee swelling.
- Healthy and balanced diet. chart
- OTC pain relievers: Ibuprofen, Naproxen, Acetaminophen.
- Cold and heat therapy. chart
- Application of compression bandage to the knee.
- Low impact activities: cycling, walking, swimming.
- Use of proper knee braces.
- Use of proper shoes for walking and sports activities.
- Arch support to the foot, if necessary.
- Yoga and meditation for mindfullness.
- In severe and acute pain, movements may be avoided.
- Healthy body weight should be maintained.
- Use of properly fitted shoes.
- Diabetes properly controlled.

When to seek medical advice:
- Pain, tenderness or, stiffness in one or more joints.
- Joints are red or warm to touch. Swollen joint.
- Joint pain that is worse after activity or at rest.
- Clicking or cracking sound from joint when joint bends.
- Difficulty in moving a joint or doing daily life activities.

Low Back Pain.

If you rest, you rust.

Spine or, back bone

Spine or back bone is the central support structure of the body. The spine is made up of small bones, called vertebrae. Vertebra are stacked on top of one another and create the natural curve of the back. In between two vertebra, vertebral discs are situated. Vertebral discs are rounded, flat rubbery pads filled with gel like material. Vertebral discs act as a cushion and shock absorber in between each of vertebra in the spine. They provide wide range of motion to the spine.

Spine extends from the base of the skull to the tailbone. The spine encloses the spinal cord and is surrounded by muscles, tendons and other tissues.

Spinal cord is a column of nerve tissue and extends from the continuation of brain at the base of the skull down to the centre of the back.

Low back pain

Low back pain is a common disorder. It is like common cold as it affects majority of population at any age of his life time. It is an universal complain.

The pain is felt on the back of the trunk, hip, back of thigh and leg and may radiate upto the sole of the foot.

Back pain involves the muscles, nerves, ligaments, bones and other tissues of the spine. Pain may vary from a constant ache to a sudden sharp distressing feelings.

Causes of back pain:
- Pain may start without any obvious cause.
- Muscle or ligament strain caused by:
    - repeated lifting of heavy weights.
    - sudden awkward movement of back bone.

BODY PAIN AND PAIN RELIEF

- o poor physical condition, which may cause constant strain on back muscles and ligaments and cause muscle spasm.
- Bulging of disc material of backbone (spine).
- Fall from height and causing trauma to the spine.
- Infection and inflammation of bones and joints of spine.
- Osteoporosis of bones of spine makes the spine porous and brittle and causes fractures and pain.
- Tumors of any tissue of vertebral column.

Risk factors for back pain:

- After 40, back pain increases with increase of age.
- Excess body weight. Lack of exercise and body movements.
- Sedentary lifestyle with weak back muscles.
- Improper technique in lifting of weights.
- Sometimes low back pain is familial.
- Poor posture in walking, sitting and sleeping.
- Mental depression.
- Some diseases predispose LBP:
    - o Osteoporosis (porus bone).
    - o Infection, inflammation and tumors of spine.
    - o Herniated intervertebral disc (sciatica).

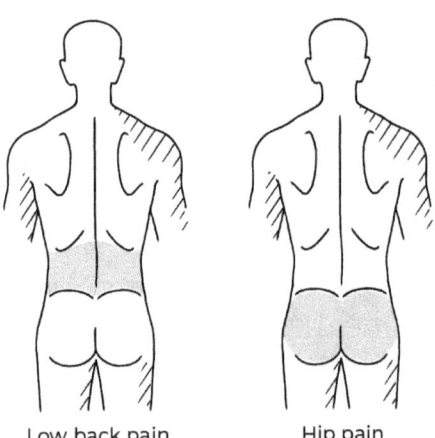

Low back pain   Hip pain

Low Back Pain.

Features of back pain:

- Intermittent or continuous back pain, that may radiate to the lower extremities and sometimes upto sole of the foot.
- Pain is dull or achy, stinging or burning.
- Back muscles feel stiff.
- Muscle weakness affect back, buttocks, legs, and feet.
- Tingling or loss of sensation from lower back to feet.
- A grinding or popping feeling on moving the spine.
- Poor co-ordination in walking with loss of balance and difficulty in walking.
- Defecation and micturation control may be in trouble.

Long term complications of back pain:

- Chronic pain and discomfort. Permanent physical disability.
- Absenteeism from work and loss of work hour.
- Weakness in the lower limb and gait gradually changed.
- Control of defecation and micturation may be disturbed.
- Quality of life is downgraded.

Prevention of low back pain:

Low back pain can be prevented to some extent by making some lifestyle changes. Long term precautions are beneficial.

Preventive measures are:

- Body weight should be kept within normal healthy range.
- Healthy and balanced diet. chart
- Must remain physically active. 'Motion is lotion' for the spine. Prolonged bed rest can actually make the condition worse.
- Habit of prolonged sitting or standing in one position should be avoided. One minute of brisk walking in every one hour of sitting is beneficial.
- Healthy and good posture for prolonged sitting, standing or lying.
- Always sit with keeping the back straight but relaxed with back support if required.
- While sitting, the chair height should be adjusted so that the knees are slightly higher than the hips. Use of a *foot rest* will help.
- Back support, distence of computer monitor and book from eye should be maintained by taking advice from expert. see neck pain, page

- Use of flat bed with firm mattress (not too hard nor too soft) and healthy posture for sleeping is beneficial. Must sleep on the side with bent knees. A side pillow between the bent knees is much beneficial.
- To get up from lying position, turn on any side first, bend the hips, knees, and take support of the upper arm.
- Weight lifting should be avoided. To lift relatively heavy objects, bend the knees and hips and keep the back straight and squat near the object. Keep the object close to the body and slowly stand by straightening the knees and hips keeping the back straight.
- Never bend at the waist keeping the knees straightened. If it is necessary to bend the waist, first bend the knees then bend at the waist. This maneuver will prevent over stretching of the nerve (sciatic nerve) and back pain.
- Do not read papers or magazines in lying position with too many pillows under the head.
- Stooping forward (bending at the waist) should be avoided. Washbasin of correct height should be used.
- Do not try to reach for heavy objects overhead.
- Frequent bending and twisting of spine must be avoided.
- Use car seat with lumbar support.
- Long drive in a bad road is injurious to spine.
- Donot ride vehicles for very long distence at a stretch.
- Avoid sudden and jerky movements of the body.
- Sufficient good sleep.
- Management of depression.
- Smoking avoided.

Home remedies for back pain:

- Follow the preventive measures.
- Maintenance of healthy body weight. chart
- Healthy and balanced diet.chart
- Try to keep moving. Remember 'Motion is lotion'. Usual level of daily activities and movements are continued.
- Stretching and strengthening exercises for the back and abdominal muscles are practised.
- Use of heating pack will relieve stiff and achy muscles.
- OTC cream use: Ketoprofen, Ibuprofen, Diclofenac.
- Use of well-fitted shoe.
- Maintenance of good posture in bed and in chair.

Low Back Pain.

- Must sleep on the side with bent knees and a side pillow in between the bent knees.
- Sufficient good sleep and reduction of mental stress.
- Movement therapies such as Yoga and tai-chi. These can help to stretch and strengthen the back muscles.
- Swimming in a warm pool. Warm pool exercises.
- Therapeutic body massage: chart
- OTC pain relievers: acetaminophen, ibuprofen, naproxen.
- Weight-lifting should be strictly avoided.

Correct posture for lifting of weights.

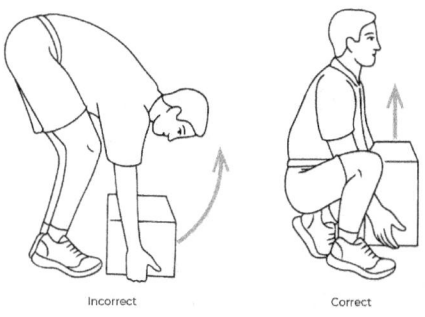

Proper lifting

- Weight lifting must be avoided.
- If it is a situation for domestic requirement, please do not try to lift object that are awkward or are heavier than 10 kg.
- Before holding the object, a firm footing is ensured and then start the action.
- To pick up an object that is lower than the level of the waist, the back should be kept straight and knees and hips are bent and sit close to the object with a wide stance.
- Please do not bend forward at the waist with the knees keeping straight.
- Feet should be firm on the ground. Belly muscles are tightened and the object is lifted using the leg muscles. Knees and hips are straightened in a steady motion. Never to jerk the object up to the body.

- Complete upright posture is maintained during standing and no twisting of the trunk is allowed. Always move feet forward when lifting a heavy object.
- On the occasion of lifting an object from a table-height, the object should be slided to the edge of the table so that the object can be held close to the body. Knees are bent so that the object is more closer. The object is kept closer by bending the arms. Legs are used to lift the object and come to a standing position. Belly muscles are kept tight. Take small steps and go slowly.
- Lifting of heavy object above waist level should be avoided.
- To lower the object, first feet are placed firm as it is done during lifting. The belly muscles are tightened and the hips and knees are bent and the object is lowered. Never to bend forwards at the waist.

Walking and back pain.

Walking is an effective approach for relieving back pain. Regular walking increases the release of *endorphins*. Endorphins are chemicals produced by the body in response to walking, exercise, other physical activities like sex, pain and stress. They relieve pain and stress.

Walking tips:
- Back should be kept in neutral position. Head is positioned on the top of the spine with the ears above the shoulders.
- Steps of walking should be taken in such a way that the foot lands on the ground and touches the ground between the mid-foot and the heel and then gently roll onto the toes. Push-off done to progress to the next step.
- Shorter and slower steps are beneficial.
- Support using a walking stick may be helpful.
- Incorrect walking posture can compress the spine and increase the back pain.
- Toe should not be used during walking. Only mid-foot and heel should be used. This will shorten the steps and slow down the walking speed.
- During walking in correct posture, the following muscles will work in sync and prevent stress on the spine and relieves pain. The muscles are:
  o Back muscles. Abdominal muscles.
  o Muscles of the hip. Muscles of thigh, and
  o Leg muscles.
- During walking, breaks should be taken for a few moments frequently and deep breathing exercise is practiced.

Low Back Pain.

- Stretching exercises for the leg, thigh and back muscles should be done daily and regurlarly.

Avoid:

- High-impact-sports, exercises and movements that strain the back muscles.
- Any posture, movement, and exercise that cause pain.

Benefits of good walking posture:

Maintaining proper walking posture is very beneficial for back pain and neck pain.

Benefits of walking: chart

Posture and spine health

Posture is the position in which someone holds their body while standing, sitting or lying down. The position of the spine is the key to good posture. The spine has three natural curves. They are in the *neck, mid back* and *low back*. Correct posture should maintain these curves.

Good posture involves exercising the body to stand, walk, sit and lie so as to impact the least strain on supporting muscles and ligaments while moving or performing weight-bearing activities.

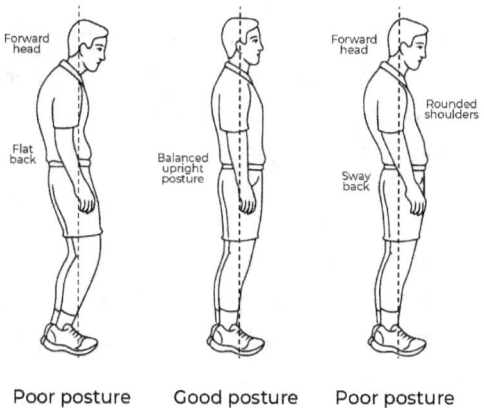

© Dr. Abu Hena Mahboob

BODY PAIN AND PAIN RELIEF

Good posture keeps bones and joints in the correct alignment so that muscles are being used properly, prevents or delays wear and tear of joint surfaces and thus prevent the onset of arthritis. Reducing strain on the ligaments and muscles in the spine, delay the onset of back pain and muscular pain. Muscle fatigue is prevented as muscles are used more efficiently. Less energy is required for daily life activities.

Good posture for *standing*:

- Ears lined up with the centre of the shoulder. Shoulders should be kept back.
- Shoulders align with hips. Hips align with ankles.
- Body weight distributed evenly in both feet. Put body weight mostly on the balls of feet.
- Ears, chin, shoulders, hips and feet will be in the same horizontal plane.
- Feet should be kept about shoulder-width apart.

Good posture for *sitting*:

- Ears lined up with the centre of the shoulder. Back should be straight and shoulders turned back. The trunk should be drawn up. All three normal back curves should be present while sitting. A small, rolled-up towel or a lumbar roll may be used to help to maintain the normal curves in the back.
- Elbows, hips and knees are bent at 90^0. Knees may be kept slightly higher than the hips. Footrest or a stool may be used.
- Never to cross the legs in sitting posture.
- Buttocks should touch the back of the chair.
- Body weight should be distributed evenly on both hips.
- It is better to avoid sitting in the same position for more than 30 minutes.
- At work, the chair height and the desk height should be adjusted, so that the distance from the eye is proper. Elbow, arm and shoulder should be kept relaxed.
- If the chair rolls and pivots, it is better not to twist at the waist while sitting. Body as a whole should be turned.
- On standing from the sitting position, first move to the front of the chair. Stand up by straightening the legs. Bending forward at the waist should be avoided. Back stretching is beneficial.

Good posture for *sleeping* and *lying down*:

The following recommendations will benefit most of the people who have back pain. If any of these guidelines cause increase of pain or the pain spreads to the legs, the activities should be stopped and advice from a physician or a physical therapist may be seeked.

- The mattress should be firm that does not sag.
- It is better to lie in right or left lateral position or in supine position (lying horizontally with the face and torso facing up). During lying in lateral position, knees should be kept bent with a side pillow in between the knees. During lying in supine position, a pillow should be under the head, but not under the shoulders. The thickness of the pillow will allow the head to be in a neutral position, another pillow may be placed under the leg to make the knees slightly bent. This position will reduce tension to the nerve (sciatic nerve) and reduce pain.
- A lumbar support may be used when lying in supine position.

Get-up from lying position.

- For standing up from the lying position, body should be turned to one side, both knees are drawn up and the legs are swinged on the side of the bed. Sit up by pushing the body up with hand. Bending forward at the waist should must be avoided.

Back pain and food habits

Foods to *avoid* while suffering from back pain:

- *Sugary foods.* These are the worst.
  - Honey, Glucose, Dextrose drink. Fruits juices.
  - Sweetened tea, coffee, chocolate milk.
  - Sports drinks, energy drinks. sweet yogurt.
- *Vegetable oils:* oils rich in omega-6 fatty acids.chart
- *Refined grains:* white breads, refined rice, pizza.
- *Dairy products,* Red meat, Fatty foods. Processed foods.
- Foods with *artificial sweetner* and *coloring agents.*
- Foods with monosodium glutamate (MSG).
  - Fast foods, chinese foods. Processed meat.
  - Chips and snack foods, salad dressings.
  - Instant noodle products. Frozen meals. Soups.

BODY PAIN AND PAIN RELIEF

- *Preserved foods:* These are packaged, refrigerated, frozen, canned and dried foods. Gluten containing foods.
- Peanuts, tomatoes, Caffeine, Chocolate.

Beneficial foods in back pain:

- *Plant* based proteins: Lentils, edamame, peanuts, chickpeas, spirulina, tofu, almonds, legumes, beans, pulses.
- *Leafy Green vegetables:* chart
- *Nuts and seeds:* walnut, almonds, pecan, chia seeds.
- *Fresh fruits:* avocados, cherries, grapes, pomegranates.
- *Lean protein:* chicken, turkey, fish.
- *Sea foods:* Tuna, salmon, mackerel, sardins, shellfish.
- *Olive* oil, olive. Fish oil. Turmeric, ginger.
- Calcium and vitamin D suppliments.

When to seek medical advice:

- Back pain accompanied by fever.
- Pain accompanied by weakness, tingling or numbness in the legs and feet. Pain following trauma to the spine.
- Pain lasts longer than six weeks. Pain causing sleep disturbance.
- Pain that gets worse even after at-home treatment.
- Pain is associated with micturation and defecation trouble.

Low back pain in elderly people: See page

Menopause and Body Pain

'There is no more creative force in the world than the menopausal womenwith zest'

—Margaret Mead.

Menopause means stoppage of menstruation. It is the period that marks the permanent cesation of menstrual activity. Normally menopause occurs between the ages of 40 and 60. Menopause is said to have occured once the women has experienced 12 full months without any menstrual bleeding. The mean age is 50. Age may vary in different areas of the world. The menses may stop suddenly, but this phenomenon is relatively rare and generally total stoppage occurs gradually. Menopause is associated with a natural decline in estrogen hormone. Estrogen helps to reduce inflammation in the body.

Decline in estrogen will cause increase in visceral fat mass, decrease in bone mass density, and decrease in muscle mass and strength. Estrogen deficiency also increases inflammatory activities and pain in the body.

Menopause causes body pain by affecting different structures of the body. The pain increases as the menopause period progresses.

Menopause and body pain can be discussed under the following headlines:
- Muscle pain. Joint pain.
- Menopause related joint inflammation.
- Osteoporosis (porous bone).
- Headache. Fibromyalgia.

Muscle pain

Muscle pain is commonly experienced during menopause and can range from a mild discomfort to chronic pain. Natural aging process is usually ascribed to aches and pains. The hormonal changes in the body which occurs during the menopause is also responsible for pain and tender feeling of muscles. These aches and pains are commonly experienced in the back, shoulders and neck. Tension headache which occurs in menopause is also caused by hormonal changes. Pain may occur all over the body and can disrupt sleep.

As menopause starts, the hormonal imbalance is the most common reason for muscle aches and pain. The imbalance of estrogen and progesterone and cortisol are the main causes. The estrogen and progesterone are the principal female hormones.

Estrogen helps to reduce inflammation. Estrogen regulates the production of cortisol in the body. Cortisol is a 'stress hormone'. When estrogen production is low, the secretion of cortisol will rise. Cortisol will cause more stressed and anxious. These two symptoms are very common in the menopausal period. High levels of cortisol can cause muscles to tense up and painful. Cortisol also increases the sensitivity of pain fibers. As a result of increased sensitivity, patient will feel muscle and body aches and pains more intensely.

Low estrogen can also affect the uptake and utilization of magnesium. Magnesium is vital for proper muscle function and muscle relaxation. So,low magnesium will cause muscle aches and pains, muscle fatigue and muscle cramps.

Progesterone is a hormone which keeps the body in harmony and relaxed. During menopause, the level of progesterone is dropped and causes muscle tension and pain.

Hormonal and physical changes during the menopause can also cause weight gain and develop fat around the waist and buttock. The increased weight can put more strain on muscles and joints, resulting in pain in joints and discomfort in the body.

Anemia in menopause also cause lack of oxygen supply in the muscles causing muscular ischaemia and pain.

Home remedies:

Regular gentle exercises: walking, cycling, swimming.

- Stretching exercise to reduce stiffness and muscle pain.
- Healthy and balanced food intake. chart

- Anti-inflammatory foods: chart
- Avoidence of foods causing inflammation: chart
- Vitamin and mineral supplements.
- Warm water bath.
- Massage: deep tissue massage will increase blood circulation, reduce toxin built-up and soothe muscle pain, tension and stiffness. It can also promote relaxation and reduces stress. chart
- Maintaining healthy body weight. chart
- Sufficient water intake to make body hydrated. chart

Joint pain

Joint pain is one of the most common symptom of menopause. Joints which are involved in high impact movements such as the hips, knees, ankles and feet are tend to be most affected. The elbows, neck, shoulders, hands and fingers can also be affected by joint pain.

Causes of joint pain during menopause:

- Hormonal changes in the body.
- Dehydration. Weight gain.
- Anxiety and mental stress.
- Faulty diet.
- Poor posture in the bed,chair.
- Increased sensitivity to pain.

Falling estrogen level is one of the main cause of joint pain during menopause. Estrogen is responsible for regulating fluid levels in the body. When estrogen level is low, the body becomes less able to hold water and affect the hydration and lubrication of the joint tissues including the cartilage, ligaments and tendons. Water is also needed to help to support the flexibility and elasticity of the ligaments and tendons. When ligaments and tendons lose their elasticity, range of movement of joints will be reduced. It will also cause aches, pains and stiffness to develop.

Flactuating estrogen levels may also give rise to low-grade inflammation and joint pain. Estrogen is an anti-inflammatory agent.

Low estrogen will increase the stress hormone, cortisol. Cortisol acts as an anti-inflammatory agent, but increased cortisol will increase stress and increased stress will cause muscles to tense- up. This tension will cause increase in workload to the joint and leads to discomfort and pain.

Weight gain is a common problem during menopause and is caused by increased cortisol in the body. Excess weight puts additional pressure on weight-bearing joints such as the knees, hips and ankles and causes joint trauma and pain.

Level of magnesium is an important factor. Poor levels of magnesium is very common during menopause due to stress and digestive weakness. Magnesium is needed to keep muscles relaxed. So, low level can cause the muscles to tense up and become tight and stiff and joint movement will be difficult.

Menopause related joint inflammation (arthritis) and pain are also important factors. Menopausal joint inflammation can run in family. This may be due to disturbance of the metabolism of estrogen due to the presence of abnormal genes. Genes are genitically inherited. Estrogen is reduced in menopause. Estrogen has anti-inflammatory effects. As the estrogen level is reduced, inflammation may increase and cause discomfort and menopause related arthritis. Menopausal women's arthritis symptoms get worse faster.

Home remedies for joint pain:

- Maintenance of healthy body weight.
- Plenty of water intake.
- Non-weight bearing physical exercises like warm pool swimming, cycling, water aerobics in warm pool etc.
- Low-impact exercises: walking, cycling, swimming, yoga.
- Healthy and balanced diet.chart
- Food suppliments: Magnesium, Calcium, vitamines.
- OTC pain relievers: Ibuprofen, Naproxen, Acetaminophen.

Osteoporosis (porus bone) and pain

Osteoporosis means 'porous bone'. Osteoporosis results in an increased loss of bone mass and strength. Osteoporosis has a direct relationship with lack of estrogen. In menopause, there is relative lack of estrogen and cause more bone resorption than formation, resulting in osteoporosis.

Severe pain in the back is the main symptom. Sometimes pain may occur in the whole body. Loss of body height or spinal deformities such as stooped posture may be marked.

Home remedies:

- Weight- bearing physical activities are encouraged.
- Exercise: Brisk walking.
- Balanced and healthy diet.chart
- Food supplements: Calcium, vitamin D, B-complex and C.
- Foods rich in Calcium and Vitamin D.
- Smoking and alcohol should be avoided.
- Some medications according to physician advice.

Menopause and headache

Most women experience headache, particularly around the time when a period is due. It is not unusual for this symptom to reappear during the menopause as hormone levels rise and fall at this time. Menopause headaches are most common among women who have suffered from headaches before, particularly around their menstrual period.

Several types of headaches are triggered by menopause.

Migraines: These are the most intense type of headache. The pain grows generally on one side of the head or behind the eyes and begins to pulsate or throb. This is sometimes accompanied by aura or flashing lights and nausea.

Tension headaches: These may be associated with stress. They are characterized by a feeling of tightness or moderate pain across the forehead and back of the head and neck.

Sinus headache: Sinus headache is characterized by feeling of congestion in nose and experience facial pain.

The *hormones* that are affected most during the menopause are estrogen and progesterone. Estrogen is thought to cause blood vessels to dilate, while progesterone cause them to tighten. As the levels of these hormones fluctuates, the blood vessels are constantly expanding and contracting. This can cause pressure changes in the head and result in the headache.

Home remedies:

- Avoidence of certain foods: Chocolate, Caffeine, Redwine.
- Avoidence of stress and anxiety.

- Regular eating habit. Taking of small snacks frequently.
- Regular taking of balanced and healthy diet. chart
- Calcium and magnesium suppliments.
- Dark green vegetables. Dried fruits. Nuts. Whole grains.

When to seek medical advice for *menopause symptoms:*

- Symptoms of menopause develop before 45 years of age.
- Extreme symptoms interfereing activities of daily life.
- Unexpected symptomes like:
    o A lot of weight gain.
    o Dizziness.
    o Increased anxiety.
- Vaginal bleeding after menopause.
- Sexual dysfunction.
- Symptoms that disrupt the emotional, physical or mental rhythms of life.
- Control on urination and defecation are reduced.

Menstrual Cramp

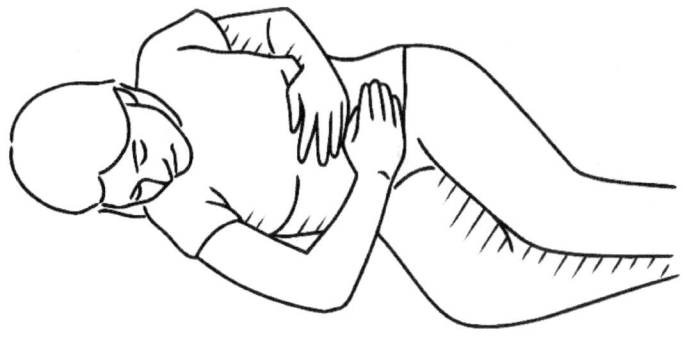

Position in menstrual cramp

Menstrual cramp is also called as period pain.

Uterus is a muscular organ. Menstrual cramp occurs because of contractions in the muscles of uterus. If uterus contracts too strongly during menstrual cycle, it can press the blood vessels and causes reduction in blood and oxygen supply to the uterus. Due to lack of oxygen, tissue necrosis (death) occurs and causes pain and cramping.

Menstrual cramps are one of the most common cause of period pain. It is an annoying part of menstrual period. Menstrual cramps can strike just before or during the time of menstrual cycle. Many women get them routinely.

Menstrual cramp can range from mild to severe. It can worsen with age and can last for the entire duration of the period.

BODY PAIN AND PAIN RELIEF

Cause of menstrual cramp:

Menstrual cramp is caused by an excess of some chemicals which act like hormones. They are released by the uterine lining as the uterus process to be shed. These chemicals help the uterus to contract and relax, and menstrual flow occurs.

Features of menstrual cramp:

- Throbbing or cramping pain in the lower abdomen. The pain may be intense in character.
- Pain starts 1-3 days before starting period, peaks 24hrs after the onset of period and subsides in 2-3 days.
- Dull, continuous ache.
- Pain may radiate to the lower back and thighs.

Home treatment for menstrual cramp:

- Life style changes.
    - Enough sleep and rest. Regular physical exercises.
    - Dietary supplementation.
    - Mind relaxation. Stress reduction.
    - Meditation and mindfullness. Yoga.
- Dietary supplementation.
    - Vitamin E. Omega-3 fatty acids. Vitamin B_1, B_6.
    - Magnesium supplementation.
- Making the body curled-up will reduce pain.
- Use of heat patch on lower abdomen.
- Massage belly with essential oils like lavender, sage, rose.
- Stay hydrated. Take plenty of water.
- OTC pain reliever: Ibuprofen, Naproxen, Acetaminophen.
- Physical exercises: walking, gogging, dancing, cycling.
- Hot bath. Soak in a warm bathtub.
- Having an orgasm.

Foods to *avoid*:

- Salty foods. Spicy foods.
- Canned food: They are high in salt. Salt causes cramp.
- Processed foods. All bakery foods. Extra salt in diet.
- Beans. Milk and dairy products. Refined sugar.

- Coffee. Chocolate. Fatty foods. Alcohol.

Beneficial foods:

- Whole grain foods. Oatmeals. Lean protein. Poultry. Eggs.
- All citrus fruits. Green vegetables.
- Dark chocolate. Chamomile tea.
- Green tea. Cinnamon. Ginger. Turmeric. Fennel extracts.

When to seek medical advice for *menstrual cramp:*

- Severe cramps. May interfere the activities of daily life.
- Pain spreads to the back and down to the thigh and legs.
- Cramp suddenly gets worse.
- Sudden, severe cramp above 25 years of age.
- Cramp is accompanied by: Fever, Heavy vaginal bleeding and chest pain.
- Periods are getting heavier and cramps are getting worse over a 2-3 months time period.
- Cramps and pain continues in between bleeding periods.
- Cramp is not relieved by OTC pain relieving drugs and home remedies.

Ovulation Pain

The best is yet to come.

Ovulation pain is normal. About one in five women experience pain during ovulation that can last from a few minutes to 48 hours. Ovulation pain is usually harmless and not a sign of a serious health condition. Ovulation pain does not affect fertility. Ovulation pain can help to be more aware of the time of ovulation. Rarely, ovulation pain may indicate various medical conditions.

Causes of ovulation pain:

- Just before an egg is released with ovulation, follicle growth stretches the surface of the ovary and causes pain.
- Blood or fluid released from the ruptured follicle irritates the lining (peritoneum) of the abdominal and pelvic cavity causing pain.

Features of *ovulation* pain:

- *Pain* in the lower abdomen and pelvis. Pain is one sided, right or left side.
- Pain typically occurs about 14 days before the next menstrual period.
- Pain is sudden, dull and achy, similar to menstrual cramp. Pain may be like uncomfortable pressure, twinges and sharp achy.
- Pain may last for few minutes to 48 hours.
- Pain may be accompanied by vaginal bleeding or discharge.

Home remedies for ovulation pain:

- Lower abdomen should be kept warm. Heat pack or hot water bottle may be used.
- Warm bath. Gentle massage. Gentle walking.
- OTC pain relievers: Ibuprofen, Naproxen, Acetaminophen.

BODY PAIN AND PAIN RELIEF

Foods to avoid:

- Salty foods and extra salts in diet.
- Canned food. They are high in salt. Salt causes cramp.
- Processed food. All bakery foods.
- Beans.
- Milk and dairy products. Refined sugar. Coffee. Chocolate.
- Fatty foods. Spicy foods. Alcohol.

Beneficial foods:

- Whole foods. Oatmeal. Lean protein. Poultry. Eggs.
- All citrus fruits. Green leafy vegetables.
- Dark chocolate. Chamomile tea. Green tea.
- Cinnamon. Ginger. Turmeric. Fennel extracts.

When to seek medical advice:

- Pain lasts longer than 3 days.
- Pain is associated with other unusual menstrual symptoms, such as heavy vaginal bleeding.

Muscle Pain

(Polymyalgia rheumatica, PMR)

Polymyalgia rheumatica (PMR) is a syndrome with pain and stiffness, usually in the shoulders, neck, upper arms and hips. PMR may occur all over the body. The pain may start as an acute attack or can occur gradually over a period. Most people with PMR *wake-up in the morning* with pain in their muscles. Sometimes pain and stiffness persists all day long.

Causes of PMR:

- Exact cause is not known.
- *Genetic* and *environmental* factors may be responsible.
- It is an age-related condition and mostly occur over the age of 65.

Features of PMR:

- Women are affected in most cases.
- Worse in the morning.
- *Pain* and stiffness usually occur on *both sides* of the body.
- Pain mostly in *shoulder and neck* but can occur in the upper arm, buttocks, hips or thighs.
- Headache and pain on touch to the scalp.
- Jaw pain. Vision problem.
- Morning stiffness is in the affected areas of body.
- Malaise: general feeling of unwell.
- Stiffness and pain may occur after being inactive for some time, mainly seen in wrist, elbows or, knees.
- Feeling of fatigue and general sickness.
- It can *affect* the ability to perform activities of daily life:
  o Getting out of bed or standing up from a chair.
  o Bathing. Combing hair. Getting dressed.
  o Social interactions, physical activities, sleep and general well-being.
- Joints swelling.

- Loss of appetite. Unexplained weight loss.
- Low grade fever.
- Depression.

Home remedies and prevention of PMR:

- Activities of daily life should be continued as much as possible.
- *Light physical exercises* are beneficial e.g, Gardening. Walking. Swimming. Cycling. Warm pool exercises. Light weight training.
- Healthy and balanced diet.
- OTC pain relievers: Ibuprofen, Naproxen, Acetaminophen.

Beneficial foods:

- Foods containing omega-3 fatty acids: chart
- Calcium and vitamin D supplements.

Foods to *avoid:*

- Refined carbohydrates. White bread and rice.
- Fried foods. Sugary drinks. Processed meats. Red meat.
- Margarine. Alcohol.

When to seek medical advice:

- Sleep disturbance.
- Severe symptoms.
- Activities of daily life is disrupted.

Neck Pain

If you have a neck, you should have a neck pain.

Neck is the part of the body between the head and the trunk. Neck supports the weight of the head and provides mobility and movement to the head.

Neck pain is an universal problem.

Almost everyone suffer from neck pain for some period in his lifetime. Very simple and minor causes are responsible for initiation of neck pain in majority of cases.

The most common cause of neck pain is a muscle strain, in which a muscle is stretched too far and tears. Neck muscle strain is typically caused by poor posture or support, such as sleeping with the neck in awkward positions. Most neck muscle injuries will feel better within a few days or weeks. Posture in chair or couch, number or height of pillow, height of chair-table or desk with computer monitor, position and height of TV screen in the room may be responsible for neck pain. But, in rare and very unfortunate cases the cause of neck pain may be life threatening. So, it is not wise to overlook neck pain initially. Care must be given to exclude any serious type of neck pain.

Neck is formed by many bones (vertebrae), muscles, joints, ligaments, blood vessels and nerves.

Neck pain is the pain that starts in the head or neck region and can be associated with radiation of pain down in the shoulder and in one or both of the arms, forearms, hands and fingers.

Neck pain may come from a number of disorders or diseases that involves any tissue in the neck and head area.

Many a times neck pain starts without any obvious reason and pain relieves spontaneously without any treatment.

Common *causes* of neck pain:

- Age: Neck pain can occur at any age but, as age increases, the joints worn-out and osteoarthritis of the neck joints will cause pain.
- Sprain and strain of ligaments and muscles of neck.
- Trauma to neck by road traffic accident: whiplash injury etc.

Whiplash injury: whiplash is the flexible part of a whip. whiplash is a neck injury due to forceful, rapid back-and-forth movement of the neck, like the cracking of a whip. Whiplash is commonly caused by a rear-end car accident, sports injury, physical assault and fall from a height. Generally, whiplash is like a neck sprain or strain injury. Whiplash injury may lead to chronic neck pain and many other long-standing complications.

- Heavy weight bearing on the head.
- Nerve compression in the neck area.
- Faulty use of chair-table, desk for reading, desk work, computer use etc. Level of book and computer monitor in relation to eye level is very important.
- Poor posture in bed.
- Mental anxiety, tension and depression.
- Uncontrolled high blood pressure and diabetes mellitus.
- Diseases of the neck:
  - Osteoarthritis.
  - Rheumatoid arthritis.
  - Ankylosing spondilitis.
  - Malignancy of any tissue in the neck.
- Diseases of head region:
  - Meningitis. Enchephalitis. Brain tumors.
- Smoking.

Risk factors and aggravating factors for neck pain:

- Women are more affected than men.
- New sprain of neck muscles or ligaments.
- Poor posture of neck during sleeping, sitting, standing, walking, reading, writting, watching TV etc.
- Poor computer workstation design and work.

- Unaccustomed use of neck.
- Neck injury in contact sports, injury from a fall or whiplash injury to the neck.
- Motor vehicle injury.

Features of neck pain:

- Can occur at any age. Women are more affected than men.
- Pain starts on working in a constant position for a long time:
  o Reading/writing.
  o Driving car.
  o Working at a computer.
- Feeling of tightness and spasm in the neck.
- Persistent pain in the neck. Pain increases on movement of the neck. Pain is stabbing or burning in nature.
- Pain may spread to the shoulder, arm, hand and fingers.
- Movement range of head is gradually decreased or inability to move the head to sides due to muscle spasm.
- Tingling, numbness and weakness in hands and feet.
- Neck pain is associated with headache.
- Quality of life is reduced.

Features which indicate a serious health problem:

- Neck pain associated with headache, stiffneck and fever.
- Pain gradually increased in intensity even after taking treatment at home.
- Tingling, numbness and weakness in hands and feet and these symptoms gradually increases.
- Pain spreads in both upper and lower limbs.
- Neck pain starts after a fall from height, road traffic accidents or any other trauma.
- Neck pain with unexplained nausea, vomiting, drowsiness, confusion, mood swings, weight loss.
- Neck pain with micturation and defecation problems.

Prevention of neck pain:

- Yoga and mind relaxation.
- Frequent change of posture and position. Never to stand or sit in one position for a too long period.
- Neck stretching from time to time.

- Maintenance of *healthy posture:*

  When in sitting position
  - Seat should be firm, not too hard nor too soft.
  - Crossing the legs on sitting posture should be avoided.
  - Feet should be kept over a footrest. Knees should be at or above the level of hips.
  - Shoulders should be parallel to the floor.
  - Head should be over the shoulder, in neutral position, not forward, backward or even to the side.
  - Chair with handrest is better.

  When in standing position
  - When standing for a long time, body weight should be shifted from one foot to another frequently. One knee should be slightly bent.
  - Feet should be at shoulder distance apart.
  - Head should be over the shoulder, in neutral position, not forward, backward or even to the side.

  When lying down in bed
  - Better lying positions are on right or left side or on the back.
  - On lying on back, a rounded pillow under the neck and another pillow under the knees to make the knees slightly bent, is better to support the natural curve of the neck.
  - On side lying posture, the spine should be kept straight by using a pillow that is higher under the neck than the head. A pillow should be kept in between the knees. The knees are kept slightly bent.
  - Sleeping on the stomach in prone position is worst.
  - Firm mattress use is essential. Mattress should be neither too hard nor too soft.
  - Too high or stiff pillow must be avoided.

  During walking
  - Eye sight level should be kept relatively parallel to the ground.
  - Stand up straight. Back should not be stooped or arched.
  - Leaning forward and backward should be avoided. Leaning puts an extra strain on the back muscles.
  - Eyes should look forwards. Looking down is better to avoid. Eye focus should be about 20 feet ahead.
  - Chin should be up and parallel to the ground. This reduces strain on the neck and back muscles.

- o Shoulders should be loosened and kept slightly back and relaxed. Loosening up the shoulders will help to relieve tension. Backward position of shoulders help to use arm and proper good arm motion during walking.
- o Abdominal and back muscles should be tightened, so that, they maintain good posture and resist stooping and leaning.
- o Pelvis should be kept neutral. It should not tilt forward or back during walking.

Watching TV.
- o Don't watch TV in bed.
- o Sitting place should be firm.
- o Back should be touching the chair back rest. 'Lumbar roll' or 'rolled towel' may be used behind lower back to provide support while sitting.
- o Avoid spending prolonged periods on soft couches.
- o Position of sitting should be changed on every 30 minutes on the couch, chair or floor.
- o Non-symetrical and unsupported positions should be avoided.
- o Side-lying with the head on cushion with the neck 'crooked' to side is unhealthy position and should be avoided.
- o TV should be set directly infront at mid vision height.
- o During breaks, change of posture positions and to get up and walk around may be done. Some gentle stretching for the neck muscles are also helpful.
- o If low back pain sufferers also suffer from neck pain should never be seated in a 'reclined' position with the legs extended straight in front.

Computer monitor and neck pain

Working at a unhealthy desk is a common cause of back and neck pain. Generally people accomodate himself to the unhealthy workstation instead of changing the position of workstation and computer monitor. Many people get strain to see a computer monitor that is too far away, too low, too high, too small or too dim. All these situations compromises good posture.

BODY PAIN AND PAIN RELIEF

Tips for computer monitor placement.

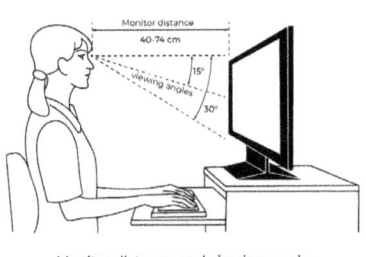

Monitor distance and viewing angle

Table - chair for monitor use

- Healthy and good posture should be maintained by adjustment of monitor height and keyboard placement.
- The chair should recline at least 25 to 30⁰ allowing to lean back. Good lumbar support will keep the back arched and the back should flush against the chair. Neck should be positioned so that the head would fall backward instead of forward if fall in asleep. Finally, feet should be placed flat on the floor.
- Computer screen should be directly in front so that no twisting or turning the body, even slightly, to see the full screen is needed.
- Eyes should look slightly downward when viewing the middle of the screen. The center of the screen should be around 15-20⁰ below the eye level. Monitor position should be at least 20 inches or 51 cm from the eyes. If the screen is larger, distance will be greater.
- Never to look up or too far down at the computer screen. If the screen is up and need to look up, the head tilts backwards and if the screen is too low the neck will go forwards. Both positions can cause strain in the neck and shoulders and pain in those areas.
- If the monitor is not of right height, It should be moved to right height.
- In case of more than one monitor, the main one should be directly infront and others by the side. Revolving chair will help.
- Frequent walk around during prolonged working period is helpful. One minute of walking in every one hour and standing from the seat in every 30 minutes is beneficial.

Reading book and neck pain

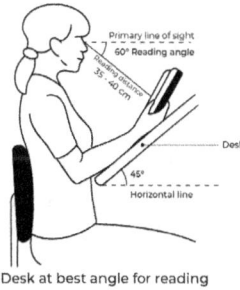
Desk at best angle for reading

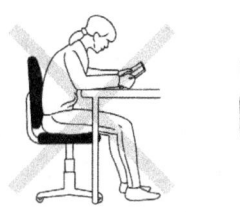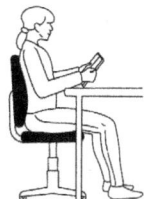
Reading table - chair

- Sitting on a chair and maintaining an upright posture with a back support pillow is ideal. The book should be held straight infront so that, the neck lean down or forward is not required to see the book. Neck should be in neutral position, that is, the head should be just above the shoulder. A small neck pillow or collar type pillow will allow proper posture and help to keep the eyes straight forward. Proper lighting on the book is a must.
- If must read in bed, sit up straight and use of a specially designed wedge pillow to prop-up the book and support for the arms may be used.
- Lying down on side with neck straight and holding the book infront may also be practiced.
- The best position in bed to read is to be in bed in supine in a firm bed. The bed should neither be too hard nor too soft to keep the spine straight and well supported. A firm neck support pillow is beneficial.
- Never to stay in one position for too long period. Change of posture in every 30 minutes is good.
- Ideal reading distence is about 35 to 40 cm or, 15 to 16 inches. It is the distence between the eyes and the book page. Ideal reading angle is 60^0.
- The best way to relax the eyes is to take a break after every 30 minutes to reduce the strain and pressure on the eyes.
- Wearing proper eye glasses is mandatory. This simple measure can prevent neck and shoulder pain and headache.

BODY PAIN AND PAIN RELIEF

Mobile phone use and neck pain

- Use of mobile phone device for prolonged period can lead to poor posture of neck and head and can result in neck and head pain.
- Looking down at the phone or tilting the head to one side during talk can lead to upper back and neck pain. Sometimes the pain ranges from a chronic, nagging pain to sharp, severe upper back muscle spasms, neck and shoulder pain and tightness in the shoulder.
- When texting on a phone, it is common to bend the head forward and look down at a 45 to 60º angle. This posture leads to stress on the neck. The neck is not able to wihstand this amount of stress over a prolonged period. This posture can also increase pressure over the surrounding nerve fibers and pain.

Prevention:

- Avoid leaning the head to one side.
- The handset should be raised up closer to the eye level, so that the head does not have to be tilted sideways and forward.
- A headset, earbuds, or speaker phone are good options to help to keep the head in a neutral position.
- Frequent breaks during talk is beneficial.
- Stretching exercises for the neck are a good practice.

When riding in a plane, train, car or, even during watching TV, a horse-shoe shaped pillow can support the neck and prevent the head from dropping to one side if doze.

Sleeping on stomach in prone position is worst, It is tough to the spine, because the back is arched and neck is turned to the side.

It is better to start the night sleeping on back or side in a well supported healthy position.

- Avoid carrying of heavy weight in the hand, on shoulder and head.
- Control of high blood pressure and diabetes.
- Avoidence of smoking.

Home remedies for neck pain:

- Rest in bed in ideal posture for a few days.
- Rest to the neck muscles during acute attack by using firm cervical collar. Use of cervical collar during travelling.
- Use of single, firm and low pillow. Use of neck pillow.
- Use of ice pack in neck in acute and severe neck pain.
- Use of heating pad or hot massage for long standing pain.
- OTC pain relievers: Ibuprofen, naproxen.
- Simple and gentle stretching of neck muscles and neck exercises should be done frequently following physician advice.
- Maintenance of healthy posture for sitting, sleeping, working, lying, standing, walking, reading and at rest.
- Adjustment of chair-table for reading-writing, computer monitor and desk for working.
- Maintennce of healthy body weight. chart
- Healthy and balanced diet. chart
- Avoidence of carrying of heavy bags in the shoulder.
- Avoidence of other aggravating factors.

When to seek medical advice:

- Neck pain is so bad that it interferes with normal activities of daily life.
- Neck pain is accompanied by fever, headache and neck stiffness. This triad of symptoms might indicate bacterial meningitis. Bacterial meningitis is an infection of the spinal cord and brain covering that requires prompt treatment with antibiotics.
- Neck pain persists after several weeks of home care.
- Neck pain worsens in spite of home care.
- Pain radiates down the arms, hands or legs.
- Neck pain is accompanied by headache.
- Neck pain causing sleep disturbances.
- Neck pain is accompanied by tingling, numbness and weakness in the arms,hands and legs.
- Loss of bowel or bladder control.
- Persistent swollen neck glands.
- Neck pain with chest pain or feeling of squeezing pressure in the chest.It may indicate heart problem.

BODY PAIN AND PAIN RELIEF

Immediately go to the *emergency room* when neck pain is accompanied by the following features:

- Fever or chills.
- Severe persistent headache. Nausea and/or vomiting.
- Sensitivity to light.
- Irregular heart beat.
- Difficulty in breathing.
- Weakness in limbs.
- Pain in the chest, jaw.
- Rash in the skin.

Osteoarthritis (OA) and Joint Pain

Being able to walk pain-free is a blessing. Being able to walk without showing the pain is a skill.

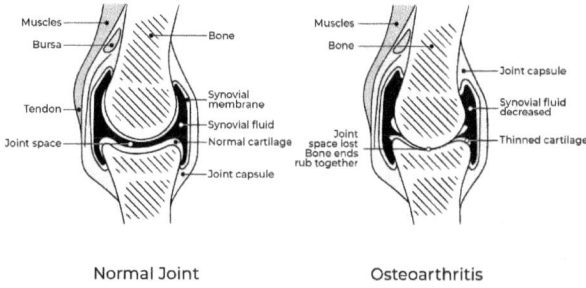

Normal Joint   Osteoarthritis

Osteoarthritis is the most common form of inflammation of joints. Generally it is a disease of older age group and affects the weight bearing joints like the spine, hip, knee, ankle and foot. Osteoarthritis symptoms can usually be managed but the damage to the joint once occur can't be reversed. So, early diagnosis and proper management can slow the progression of the disease and can improve pain and joint function.

Inflammation of joint is called arthritis.

Osteoarthritis is a type of arthritis which is marked by progressive cartilage destruction and inflammation in synovial and vertebral joints.

Osteoarthritis is the most common form of arthritis. Osteoarthritis affects millions of people worldwide every year and is a major cause of disability in older people.

Bone ends which are forming a joint are covered by a special variety of cartilage called *joint cartilage*. This cartilage forms a protective cushion at the bone ends forming the joint. Cartilage is insensitive because it has no nerve fibers. Cartilage allows painless movement of bones in a joint.

In osteoarthritis, the articular cartilage covering wears down as age increases and by many other factors. As the protective cartilage is gradually lost, underlying bone, which is sensitive to friction is exposed and movement of bones in a joint will cause pain. So, osteoarthritis is also called 'wear and tear' arthritis.

In OA, the synovial membrane forms some chemicals called cytokines, which sometimes are injurious to the joint cartilage. They cause some changes in the joint cartilage.

The changes are:
- Softening and swelling of articular cartilage.
- Fragmentation and fissuring of cartilage.
- Erosion of cartilage down to the underlying bone, and
- Exposure of underlying bone.

As bone contains sensitive nerve fibers, friction between bone ends during joint movements will cause pain.

Risk factors which are responsible for the development of osteoarthritis:

Osteoarthritis has no single cause. Combinations of several different risk factors are responsible.

Major risk factors are:
- *Genetics:* may run in families.
- *Older age:* as age increases, the incidence of OA increases.
- *Diabetes* mellitus.
- *Gender:* more in post-menopausal women.
- Over weight and obesity: strong risk factor. More body weight will cause more friction and more cartilage loss and more pain in OA.

- *Diet:* deficiency of vitamin C,D and K. Unhealthy diet.
- Previous *injury* to a joint and joint cartilage damage.
- *Congenital* abnormality of joint shape and size.
- Muscle *weakness* following a prolonged and uncontrolled diabetes, nerve and muscle injury, nerve and muscle abnormality will cause joint instability and OA.
- Some occupational factors: *porters, working in standing position like waiters, guards.*

Features of osteoarthritis:

- *Pain* in the affected joint. The nature and severity of pain is variable.
- *Swelling* of the joint.
- Joint *stiffness* (feeling tightness). Stiffness occurs after a period of inactivity.
- *Tenderness* of joint. Pressure over the joint cause pain.
- Loss of joint flexibility: range of movement of joint is reduced.
- Grating sensation: when the joint is moved a popping or crackling sound may be heard.
- Bone spurs may be formed around the affected joint.
- Feeling of fatigue and weakness.
- Reduced functional ability and activities.
- Mental depression.

Long term effects of osteoarthritis:

- Pain persists for a long time. Constantly recurring pain.
- Rapid and complete breakdown of cartilage results in the formation of loose tissue material within the joint.
- Stress fracture in the adjacent bones.
- Bone death.
- Joint pain and stiffness can become severe enough to make daily life activities very difficult.
- Sleep disturbances.
- Anxiety and Depression.

BODY PAIN AND PAIN RELIEF

Life style changes and home remedies for OA:

- Stay *active* as much as possible. Personal activities of daily life should be done by self.
- Daily *exercises:* low impact exercises:
    - walking, bicycling.
    - warm pool swimming, warm water aerobics.
    - yoga and meditation. Tai chi.
- Maintenance of healthy *body weight.*
- Healthy and balanced *diet*.chart
- Stretching *exercises.*
- *Massage* therapy.
- *Hot* and *cold* compression may relieve pain.
- Use of proper *splints* and *braces* according to physiotherapist advices.
- OTC pain relievers: Ibuprofen, Naproxen, Acetaminophen.
- Use of *shoe inserts* when necessary.
- Use of *assistive devices.* Assistive devices relieves stress on the joints:
    - *Walking stick.* Stick should be held in the hand opposite the leg that hurts.
    - Use of *gripping and grabbing tools.* These tools will make easier to work in the kitchen if OA in the fingers.

Massage therapy for osteoarthritis.

In osteoarthritis (OA), the muscles around the painful joints undergo spasm. Spasm will cause pain on movement of the joint. Muscle spasms can be smoothed using massage therapy. Massage can stimulate blood flow to the muscles and make stressed area to become more warm and relaxed. Water based exercise in a heated pool is very much effective.

Prevention of osteoarthritis:

- Maintenance of healthy body weight.
- Control of diabetes.
- Physical activities and exercises: low impact exercises are beneficial. Prevention of injuries to joints.
- Proper pain management. OTC pain reliever drugs are first tried. If not relieved, advice from physician is better.
- Management of occupational risks. Repetitive stress on the joints should be avoided.
- Healthy and balanced diet. chart

- Enjoying a rest in between work. Sufficient sleep.
- Staying positive. Abilities should be focused more rather than disabilities.

Prevention of pain in osteoarthritis:

- Body weight should be kept within normal limits.
- Control of diabetes and hypertension.
- Maintenance of active life: Exercise is a good way to prevent joint problems.
- Prevention of injury to the joint.
- Proper management for pain.Regular physical exercise.
- Maintenance of healthy lifestyle.
- Healthy and balanced diet.chart
- Adjusting workouts and day-to-day activities.

Osteoarthritis and food. See page: knee pain 258

Supplements for osteoarthritis:

- Fish oil. Glucosamine and chondroitin.
- Vitamin C,D and K supplimentation.

When to seek medical advice:

- Pain, tenderness (pain on touching the area) or stiffness in one or more joints. These symptoms are especially seen in the morning or after taking rest.
- Even after taking home remedies, gradual worsening of joint pain. Pain is seen particularly in the large weight- bearing joints of the body like hips, knees, lower back and ankles. Pain is more marked after prolonged walking or activities.
- Joints become swollen especially after walking or activities.
- Limited range of movements of joints (stiffness) in the begining of activities and stiffness goes away gradually after movements.
- Bending and straightening of joint is not complete.
- Clicking or cracking sound comes from the joint when the joint bends.
- Activities of daily life is hampered and quality of life is lowered.

Ankylosing Spondylitis (AS)

Everyday is a fight.

Ankylosing spondylitis (AS) is an inflammatory disease. It is a type of joint inflammation (arthritis) that causes mainly long term lower back pain. Pain and stiffness in the lower back and hip that may come and go. The pain is dull aching. Ankylosing spondylitis may affect almost all joints in the body, eyes, lungs, kidneys, heart, etc. It is a life long disease.

In the spine, the disease starts at the junction of the base of the spine (sacrum) and the pelvis (sacroiliac joints). As the disease progresses, new bone formation may fuse the bones of the spine. Calcium salts are deposited in the soft tissues around the spine and makes the spine more stiff. Movements of spine is greatly reduced. The pain and stiffness is felt better with movements and worse with rest.

There is no cure for ankylosing spondylitis. Life style changes can prevent the disease aggravation.

Causes and risk factors for ankylosing spondylitis:
- Exact cause of the disease is not known.
- Some genetic factors may be involved.
- May run in families.
- Men are two or three times more likely to get the disease than women.
- Mental and physical stress.
- Some bacterial (klebsiella) infection may predispose.
- Sedentary life style.
- Poor posture in sitting, walking and sleeping.
- Over weight and obesity.
- Too much strain in the back and joints.
- Sleeplessness.
- Smoking.

BODY PAIN AND PAIN RELIEF

- Chronic physical and mental stress.

Features of ankylosing spondylitis:

- Lower back pain.
- Pain and stiffness in the spine and other joints in the body especially in the morning and after a period of inactivity.
- Changes in the spine:
    o Loss of flexibility of spine.
    o Normal spinal curvatures are lost.
    o Forward leaning of the body.

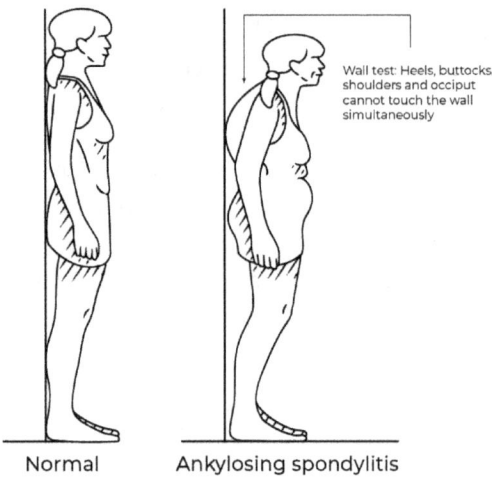

Normal   Ankylosing spondylitis

o Wall test: The patient is asked to stand with the back to the wall. His heels, buttocks, shoulders and occiput should all be able to touch the wall simultaneously. In AS, if the straightening of the spine is diminished and body leans forward, it will be impossible.
- Multiple joints may be affected: spine, knees, hips, shoulders, rib cage are commonly affected.
- Neck and hip pain. Heel pain.
- Pain is dull in nature and seems deep seated.
- Loss of appetite and weight loss.
- Fatigue and weakness.
- Fever.

- Due to involvement of rib cage:
  - Difficulty in breathing.
  - Chest tightness.
  - Rib cage pain.
- Vision disturbance.
- Gut problems (IBD).

Home remedies and prevention of AS.

Patient may get improvement of symptoms by:

- Life style changes. Exercises. Physiotherapy, and
- Medicines: OTC pain relievers may be used first. Other medicines should be prescribed by the physician.

Life style changes:

- Sedentary life style should be avoided.
- Healthy posture for sitting, walking and sleeping should be maintained.
- Patient must be remain active as much as possible.
- Personal activities of daily life should be performed by self.
- Healthy body weight should be maintained.
- Healthy and balanced diet.chart
- Get more rest. Sufficient sleep must be ensured.
- Avoid physical and mental stress. Mind and body relaxation and distraction of mind from stressful condition will improve symptoms. Long term stressful condition will release some inflammatory chemicals in the body and worsen the condition.
- To reduce stress, problems may be shared with relatives and friends.
- Strenous work and exercises are bad for the disease.
- High blood pressure and diabetes should be controlled.
- Smoking avoided.
- Spend time in nature. Adopt a pet if it reluxes mind.
- Regular visit to physiotherapist and physician.

Exercises:

Exercises should be done after consultation with a physiotherapist and/or physician.

- Deep breathing exercises are encouraged.
- Walking, swimming, cycling, dance party may help.

- Weight lifting.
- Stretching of the spine.
- Massage therapy. chart
- Heat and cold therapy. chart
- Wall sit for improvement of posture.
- Standing leg raises to loosen tight hips.
- Chin tucks to stretch the neck.
- Shoulder roll to loose up the shoulder area.
- Plank for a stronger core.
- Pilates is beneficial for core strength and stabilization.
- Tai chi. Yoga.
- Meditation and mindfullness.

Physiotherapy:

All physiotherapy protocols should be supervised by a qualified physiotherapist.

Complications of AS:

- Gradual reduction of flexibility of spine and other joints.
- Difficulty in breathing and shortness of breath.
- Painful and stiff joints which gradually aggravates.
- Tingling, numbness and pain in the lower back, buttocks, hands and feet.
- Weakness in the legs, walking may become slow and feeling of fatigue.
- Functional capabilities of joints are gradually reduced.
- Heart disease and stroke.
- Eye and vision problems.
- Bowel and bladder control reduced or gradually lost.
- Fluid retention in the body.

Foods and inflammation. See page:

When to seek medical advice:

As soon as ankylosing spondylitis is suspected, medical advice should be followed.

Osteoporosis and Body Pain

The older you are, the greater is your risk of osteoporosis.

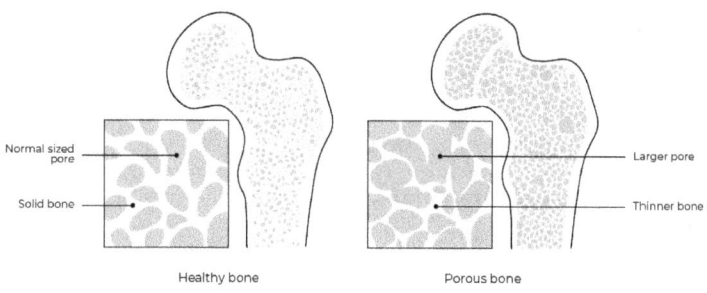

Osteoporosis

Osteoporosis means 'porous bone'. Osteoporosis is a condition of bone where the bones are weaken in quality and makes the bones more fragile and more likely to break.

Healthy bone is a living and dynamic tissue that is constantly being remodels itself. Healthy bones take up structural elements from blood and body tissues and also gives back when they are needed.

Osteoporosis is a bone disease that occurs when the body loses too much bone, makes too little bone or both.

Osteoporosis is a systemic skeletal disorder characterized by low bone mass and micro-architectural deterioration of bone tissue leading to increase in bone fragility, and consequent increase in fracture risk. As a result of osteoporosis, bones become weak and may break from a fall, minor trauma and in serious cases even from sneezing or minor falls.

Osteoporosis is a slow process and develops slowly over several years. Diagnosis of osteoporosis is incidental or occur only after a break in the bone. Mostly the patient has a history of a minor fall or sudden minor impact which causes a break. Hip, wrist and spinal fractures are most common.

Bones are thickest and strongest in early adult life until late 20s. Gradually bone losing starts from around the age of 35. This happens to everyone, but some people develop osteoporosis and lose bone much faster than normal. This means that they are at a greater risk of a fracture.

Osteoporosis itself is not always painful. When the osteoporosis is severe, it can lead to fractures at different bones and body pain. Muscle spasm occurs to support the osteoporotic bones and cause pain.

Common fractures due to osteoporosis:

- Spinal bones compression fractures.
- Hip bone fractures,and
- Wrist fractures.

Spinal compression fracture is a break of one or more small bones of the spine. In osteoporotic persons, the simple act of bending over, coughing or lifting heavy objects may cause this type of fractures. When there is more than one compression fracture, the height of the person may become shorter or the spine may be curved or humped back. Pain in the back is an important symptom.

Hip fracture in osteoporosis mostly occurs in women in old age. Fracture is generally spontaneous.

Hip fracture is marked by:

- Pain in the hip region.
- Patient can not walk or stand normally.
- Leg on the injured side looks shorter or twisted.

Wrist fractures:

This type of fractures occur due to fall on the outstretched hand. It is a common post-menopausal fracture.

Features:
- History of fall to the ground.
- Pain, swelling and bruising in the wrist or at the base of the thumb.
- Bending and deformity of the wrist.
- Gripping of objects will increase pain in hand and wrist.

Risk group people of osteoporosis:

Osteporosis can affect men and women. It is more common in older age group people, but it can occur in younger people also.

Women are more at risk of developing osteoporosis than men because the hormone changes that occur at the menopause directly affect the bone density.

The female hormone estrogen is essential for healthy bones. After menopause, oestrogen level falls. This can lead to a rapid decrease in bone density.

Women are even at greater risk of developing osteoporosis if they have an early menopause before the age of 45. Removal of the womb along with the ovaries before the age of 45 and absent periods for more than 6 months for any cause are also responsible for increased osteoporosis.

Endurance training for prolonged period in female athletes suppress menstruation and estrogen secretion and can lead to decrease in bone density and an increased risk of osteoporosis. In men, the cause of osteoporosis is unknown in most cases. Male hormone testosterone has a strong link with osteoporosis. Testosterone helps to keep the bones healthy. Men continue in producing testosterone into old age. It is documented that the risk of osteoporosis is increased in men with low levels of testosterone. In around half of men, the exact cause of low levels of testosterone is unknown. The known causes included are:
- Taking certain medicines, such as steroid use for long periods.
- Excess and prolonged alcohol intake.
- Reduced secretion of testosterone due to any cause and has abnormally low testosterone levels.

Risk factors for osteoporosis:

Many hormones in the body affect bone turnover. When there is a disorder of hormone-producing gland, there will be a higher risk of developing osteoporosis. Hormone-related disorders that can trigger osteoporosis include:

- Overactive thyroid and parathyroid glands.
- Disorders of the adrenal gland (cushing syndrome).
- Reduced amount of sex hormones, like estrogen in women and testosterone in men.
- Disorders of the pituitary gland, which is the master endocrine gland in the body.

other risk factors:

- A *family history* of osteoporosis.
- *Ethnicity.* Osteoporosis occurs in people from all ethnic groups. Europian whites and asian ancestry predisposes for osteoporosis.
- A *parental history* of hip fracture.
- A body mass index *(BMI)* of 19 or less.
- Underweight and physical inactivity.
- Long-term use of high-dose steroid.
- Prolonged use of some anti-ulcer drugs. It is due to reduced absorption of calcium in the intestine.
- Long time suffering from malabsorption and diarrhoea.
- Eating disorder like anorexia or bulimia. Malnutrition.
- Heavy smoking and alcohol consumption.
- Long term inactivity, immobilization and bed rest.
- Vitamin C, D and calcium deficiency.
- Soft drinks,which contain phosphoric acid, may increase the risk of osteoporosis, atleast in women.

Risk factors for osteoporosis which can not be changed.

Some risk factors for osteoporosis are out of control. Unchangeable risk factors are:

- *Race:* Greater risk of osteoporosis is seen in white and Asian descent.
- *Sex:* Women are much more likely to develop osteoporosis than are men.
- *Age:* Older the person, greater is the risk of developing osteoporosis both in women and men.
- *Family history:* A parent or sibling with osteoporosis has a greater risk of developing osteoporosis as grows older. If father or mother had a history of hip fracture, there will be a greater risk of developing osteoporosis and a spontaneous fracture. Sometimes a trivial injury will cause fracture.
- *Body frame size:* It is also an important factor. Men and women who have small body frames might have less bone mass and increase susceptibility to fracture.

Diseases which predispose osteoporosis:

- Long term kidney or liver diseases.
- Inflammatory bowel diseases.
- Malabsorption syndromes.
- Cancer of any organ.
- Sex hormone deficiency.
- Rheumatoid arthritis.
- Diabetes Mellitus.

Features of osteoporosis:

Osteoporosis develops slowly. A person may not know that he has osteoporosis until he experiences a fracture after a minor incident, such as a fall or without any trauma. Even a cough or sneeze can cause a break in the osteoporotic bones.

Breaks will often occur in the hip, wrist or the spinal vertebrae for people who have osteoporosis. If a break occurs in the spinal vertebrae, it can lead to changes in posture, a stoop and curvature of the spine. People might also notice a decrease in height or their cloths may not fit as well as they did previously.

Typically there are no symptoms in the early stages of bone loss. Once bones have been weakened by osteoporosis, there may have some signs and symptoms like:

- Back pain, caused by a fracture or collapsed vertebra.
- Loss of height over time.
- A stooped posture.
- A bone that breaks much more easily than expected.

Foods and osteoporosis.

Dietary factors which *increase* the risk of osteoporosis:

- Eating of foods that have a lot of common salt (sodium).
- Low calcium intake.
- Low or high animal protein intake.
- Heavy smoking. High intake of alcohol.
- Vitamin deficiency, especially vit.D_3 and vit.C.
- Eating disorder: Chronic diarrhea and malnutrition.

- Gastrointestinal surgery. Surgery to reduce the size of the stomach or to remove part of the intestine, limits the amount of surface area available to absorb nutrients, including calcium.

There are some chemicals in food that can interfere with the absorption of calcium from the gut. They are:

- *Phytic acid.* This is found in unleavened bread, raw beans, seeds and grains.
- *Oxalic acid.* This is found in spinach. The calcium that spinach contains will not be absorbed because of this oxalic acid.
- *Sodium.* High levels of sodium will interfere with calcium absorption from gut. The higher the sodium intake, the more calcium is needed to meet its daily requirements.

Foods which *prevent* osteoporosis:

Calcium and vitamin D enriched foods. See chart.

Some foods to avoid in osteoporosis, because they can *accelerate* osteoporosis:

- *Soft drinks,* even diet soda. They are packed with phosphoric acid which causes an increase in the body's acidity levels. As a result, the body will pull calcium out of the bones in order to bring the acidity levels back to normal.
- *Extra table salt.* High salt foods. *Excessive caffeine,* coffee.
- Artificially made hydrogenated oils.
- *Wheat bran. Sugary snacks.*
- Legumes. Beans. Excessive alcohol.
- Nightshade vegetables such as tomatoes, mushrooms, peppers, white potatoes and eggplant. Raw spinach.
- Excess red meat.
- Excess vitamin A.

Foods rich in calcium. See page:chart.

Foods rich in vitamin D. See page:chart

Home remedies and prevention of osteoporosis:

- Taking of healthy and balanced diet.
- Maintaining healthy body weight.
- Taking of food rich in calcium and vitamin D.

- Food supplimentation with calcium and vitamin D.
- Some foods to avoid.
- Some foods to take regularly.
- Avoidence of smoking.
- Some medications may be taken by physician advice.
- Regular physical exercises and weight-bearing activities, like:
    - Jogging. Running. Hikinng. Walking. Dancing.
    - Stair climbing. Weight lifting. Yoga. Tai chi.
    - Other aerobic exercises.

Exercises that build healthy bones:

- Foot stamps. Here one foot is put down on the ground hard and noisily and then the other foot.
- Hip-leg lifts.
- Standing on one leg alternatively.
- Repeated squat and stand.
- Biceps curls. Hamstring curls. Ball sit.

These activities help to increase bone density and make bones stronger. Cycling and swimming are not weight-bearing activities and do not help much.

Exercises to avoid in osteoporosis:

- Jumping. Jogging. Running. Climbing.
- Sudden bending forwards.
- Repeated rotating the trunk of the body.
- Golf. Hiking. Contact sports.

Home remedies for osteoporotic pain:

- Warm shower and warm pool activities. They will reduce muscle spasms and stiffness and relieves pain. chart.
- Heat and ice compression.
- Must remain physically active. Personal activities of daily living must be continued as applicable.
- Physical therapy exercises.
- Calcium, vitamin C and vitamin D suppliments.
- Use of braces and support to the limbs.
- Massage therapy. OTC pain relievers.

- There are many pharmaceutical products which are available in the market. They are effective and can prevent progression of osteoporosis. They can be used according to physician advices.

When to seek medical advice:

- Female over 50.
- Postmenopausal women.
- Body is small and thin in either sex.
- Family history of osteoporosis.
- History of taking steroids for prolonged period of time.
- History of taking medications that predispose the risk of osteoporosis.
- Suffering from diseases which predispose osteoporosis.
- Low back pain with features of osteoporosis, such as:
  - Sudden, severe back pain.
  - Back pain that gets worse on standing or walking and feels better on lying down.
  - Back pain that increases on bending or twisting.
  - Unexplained weight loss. Loss of height.
  - Gradually developing curved or stooped shape of spine with hunched posture.
  - Previous history of wrist or hip fractures.
  - Back pain is accompanied by chest pain.

Prostate Enlargement and Pelvic Pain

The prostate is a small muscular gland and is a part of male genital organs. It is located between the urinary bladder and the root of the penis. The urethra, a tube carrying urine from the urinary bladder to the exterior, runs through the centre of the prostate. The prostate secretes most of the fluid that nourishes and protects the sperm.

The muscular action of the prostate and few other structures help to propel the fluid and semen through the urethra (penis) during sexual climax.

Prostate gland enlargement is also called as benign prostatic hyperplasia (BPH). It is an universal problem for men of older age group. Enlargement of prostate occurs when the cells of the prostate gland begin to multiply. The additional cells cause prostate gland to swell and sqeeze the urethra and limit the flow of urine and it can cause symptoms that can affect the quality of life.

An enlarged prostate gland can cause uncomfortable urinary symptoms, such as blocking the flow of urine out of the urinary bladder. It can also cause urinary bladder, whole urinary tract or kidney problems.

Causes of prostate enlargement:
- It is an usual fate of aging in males. Commonly seen above the age of 60.
- Exact cause is not known.
- Male sex hormonal changes in the body as man gets older.
- Family history of prostate problems.

Features of prostate enlargement:

- Frequent urination. Urgency to urinate.
- Leakage of urine. Painful urination.
- Frequent lower abdominal and pelvic pain.

- Getting up frequently at night to urinate.
- Weak urine stream. Blood in the urine.
- An urinary stream that starts and stops.
- Dribbling at the end of urination.
- Inability to empty the urinary bladder completely.
- Straining when urinating.

Home remedies and prevention for prostate enlargement symptoms.

- Life style changes tips:
  - Choosing the healthier food options.
  - Healthy body weight should be maintained.
  - Try to remain physically active. Regular physical exercises should be done as often as possible. Walking, running, dancing, swimming, cycling are beneficial.
  - Try to stay hydrated by drinking at least 2 litres of water daily. Not to drink too much at one time.
  - Avoid drinking a lot of fluids before going out in public or starting a trip.
  - Any beverage containing alcohol and caffeine should be avoided.
  - Diabetes and hypertension should be kept controlled.
  - Urinate when get the first urge. Never delay.
  - Take time with patience to urinate to empty the bladder completely. This will reduce the need for subsequent trips to the toilet.
  - Go to the bathroom on a timed schedule, even if need to go is not felt.
  - Double void by trying to urinate again a few minutes after urinating the first time.
  - Urinate before leaving home to avoid urinary leakage in public.
  - Trying not to drink fluids in the 2 hours before bedtime.
  - Reduce or avoid stress to reduce the urge.
  - Bladder neck exercise (Kegel Exercises). Kegel exercises help to strengthen the pelvic floor muscles. Pelvic floor muscles help to control the urine flow and also control the incontinence of urine and dribbling of urine after complition of urination.

How to do Kegel exercises.
- o The exercise should be started by pulling and holding the pelvic floor muscles in for 5 seconds. To pull in the pelvic floor, the patient should think of pulling in and lifting up the genitals and forcefully close the anus.
- o After holding for 5 seconds, slowly and completely relax the muscles for 5 seconds.
- o This process should be repeated for 10 times, atleast 3 times everyday.
- Urethral massage after each urination is beneficial. Massage is done by gently pressing the fingers upwards from the base of the scrotum to try to squeeze out any urine left in the urethra and prevent any leakage later.
- Some foods to take regularly: They are:
  - o Foods containing *lycopene*. Lycopenes help to slow the progression of BPH. Lycopene cotaining foods are:
    - Tomatoes, richest source.Papaya.
    - Red cabbage, red bell peppers.
    - Guava. Carrot. Apricots.
    - Watermelon. Pink grapefruit.
  - o Foods rich in *phytoestrogen:*
    - *Soy foods, chickpeas, fava beans, alfalfa, flaxseeds, sesame seeds, oats, lentils, apples, carrots, wheat germ, whole rice.*
  - o Foods rich in *omega-3 fatty acids:* chart
  - o Foods rich in *beta-sitosterol:* Avocado.Pumpkin seeds. Wheat germ. Soybeans. Pecans.
  - o *Whole grains,* beans, legumes, dark leafy greens, broccoli, cauliflower, Kale, brussels sprouts.
  - o *Green tea. Zinc* suppliments.
  - o *Garlic. Onion. Sesame seeds. Almonds.*
- Foods to avoid:
  - o Caffeine. Artificial sweetners.
  - o Refined sugar. Excess red meat.
  - o Alcohol. Smoking. Nicotine.
  - o Carbonated drinks.

When to seek medical advice:

- Features of prostate enlargement are present.
- Gradual increase in frequency to urinate.
- Need to get up many times during night to urinate.
- Blood in the urine or in the semen.

BODY PAIN AND PAIN RELIEF

Features of prostate enlargement are accompanied by lower abdominal pain or pelvic pain and fever.

Elbow Pain

Elbow joint is one of the most complex joints in the body. One simple problem in this joint can cause complete failure of function of arm, forearm or hand. The internal make-up of this joint is much complicated.

Three bones, muscles, tendons, ligaments, blood vessels and nerves of arm and forearm jointly form the joint in such an intelligent manner that, we remain unaware of this joint and work smoothly. If any component of this joint is disturbed by any pathology, we feel pain and give attention to the area.

Normally elbow allows to extend and bend and also to rotate the forearm and hand. Since most movements are a combination of those actions, it may sometimes be difficult to describe exactly which movement brings on the pain.

Elbow pain is a very common experience. Right handed persons suffer from right elbow pain more frequently. Both right and left sides may be affected. Pain may be accompanied by swelling in the area. Lifting of even a small weight may be difficult. Pain may spread upto the shoulder and to the wrist and fingers. Twisting movements of the wrist and forearm may cause severe pain.

Pain may start with direct injury to the elbow or without any injury. Elbow pain usually is not serious, but as because, the elbow is used in so many ways, elbow pain can be very frustrating.

Causes of elbow pain:

- Excess use of hand and forearm. Repeated minor trauma will cause inflammation of the tendons (tendonitis) and cause pain.
- Repeated lifting of heavy weights will also cause inflammation of tendons and pain.
- Forceful twisting of forearm will cause sprain (tearing of some muscles, ligaments and tendon fibers) and pain.
- Inflammation (arthritis) of elbow joint. Rheumatoid arthritis. Osteoarthritis.

- Sprain and strain of tendons around the joint by forceful movements of the joint.
- Infection in elbow joint (septic arthritis).
- Infection in the bones (osteomyelitis) of elbow joint.
- Inflammed bursa (fluid filled sacs) around the joint.
- Pinched nerve in the elbow.
- Throwing injuries of elbow joint.
- Fracture of bones in the elbow.
- Dislocation of elbow joint.
- Tumour of any tissue forming the elbow.
- Uncontrolled diabetes and hypertension.

Complications of elbow pain:

- Difficult to do normal daily life activities with hand.
- Gradual restriction of range of movement of elbow.
- Movements of elbow may be stopped permanently.

Some advices to reduce elbow pain:

- Elbow may be kept in rest by using an elbow bag.
- Elevation of the elbow. Use of compression bandage.
- Use of heating pad.
- OTC pain relievers: acetaminofen, Ibuprofen, naproxen.
- If swelling is present in the elbow, elbow kept elevated.
- Use of cold and hot compression. chart

When to seek medical advice:

If pain does not relieve with home treatment for 7-10 days and the patient has the following symptoms:

- Activities of daily life is difficult due to pain in elbow.
- Pain does not relieve after taking complete rest.
- Difficulty in movements of the elbow.
- Shape of elbow is distorted.
- Pain, redness of skin, fever and swelling of elbow.

Prevention of elbow injuries:

- Over use of elbow should be avoided.
- Stretching exercise to warm-up the muscles before any sports or exercise.
- Wearing of elbow splint during sports.

Home remedies for elbow pain:

- Protection of elbow from getting further injuries.
- Avoidence of activities that cause injury to the elbow.
- Cold/hot compression in the painful area.
- Use of compression bandage to reduce swelling.
- Elevation of elbow.
- OTC pain relievers: Ibuprofen, naproxen, Acetaminofen.
- Massage of the elbow area.

If pain does not relieve after 7-10 days of home treatment, consultation with a physician will be useful.

Tennis elbow

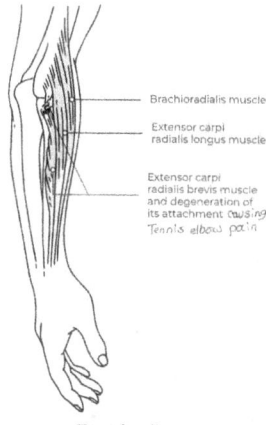

Tennis elbow

'Tennis elbow' is one of the common cause of elbow pain. There is a tiny bony bump on the outer aspect of the elbow. If the muscles of the forearm are strained by forceful activities, small tears followed by inflammation can develop near the bony bump and cause pain. Tennis elbow is mostly caused by overuse of the forearm by repetitive or strenous activity. It is the combination of frequently bending the elbow and the force placed on the arm and causes irritation in the elbow. Sometimes it may also occur after banging or knocking the elbow.

Pain is located near the bony bump and can also spread into the forearm and wrist. Pain may become severe. It may be difficult even to lift a small object. Straightening the forearm will cause severe pain.

Causes of Tennis elbow:

- Playing tennis, baseball or any other ball throwing sports.
- Manual labor. plumbing. Painting on walls and ceilings.
- Repetitive hand use, using computer mouse or typing.
- Repetitive actions involving the elbow: playing violin.

Features of Tennis elbow:

- Pain on lifting an object or bending the arm and forearm.
- Pain on twisting the forearm, arm, and even the wrist.
- Pain on gripping small objects,like pen and writing.
- Inability or difficulty in extending the forearm completely.
- Persistent pain on the outerside of the upper forearm just below the bend of the elbow and on certain occasions radiating down towards the wrist.

Home remedies and prevention for *tennis elbow:*

'Tennis elbow' pain will get better without treatment. It is a self-limiting condition. Tennis elbow usually lasts between 6 months and 2 years. The most important thing to do is to rest the elbow and to stop doing the activities those caused the pain.

- Giving rest to the arm,forearm and elbow.
- Proper use of tennis elbow brace.
- Heat compression to the outer aspect of the elbow.
- Some stretching exercises for the elbow muscles.
- OTC pain relievers: Ibuprofen, Naproxen etc.
- Massage of the part.

Heat compression in tennis elbow.

When there is severe pain, and for long-term care of tennis elbow, heat therapy is useful. Heat promotes the flow of blood to the local area by dilating small blood vessels. Heat also relaxes and expands the associated muscles and relieves pain.

Massage in tennis elbow.

Deep tissue massage to the forearm muscles, is a very effective method of relieving pain and healing of sprained muscles. Deep tissue massage will enhance the circulation and friction to the tendons will reduce local oedema and pain.

Stretching exercises:

Wrist back muscles stretching is beneficial.

When to seek medical advice:
- Home remedies do not relieve pain.
- Progressively the pain becomes worse and makes it difficult to move the arm and forearm.
- To confirm the diagnosis that, it is truely a tennis elbow.
- There is a lump or bulge in the outer aspect of elbow.

Elbow joint inflammation (arthritis)

Inflammation of elbow joint is elbow arthritis. Elbow arthritis occurs when the soft tissue is inflamed or the cartilage in the elbow becomes worn or damaged. Common causes:
- Unknown causes in rheumatoid arthritis and juvenile idiopathic arthritis.
- Older age.
- Overuse and repetitive activities of elbow joint.
- Injury: fracture or dislocation of the elbow joint.
- Osteoarthritis and gout affecting the elbow.

Features of elbow arthritis:
- *Pain* in the elbow.
- Symptoms are worse on the outer aspect of the joint.
- More pain on rotation or straightening the joint.
- Swelling of elbow.
- Feeling of stiffness in the joint during movement.
- A clicking or snapping feeling.
- Pain becomes worse on movement of the elbow joint.
- The joint may catches or locks or gives out on movement.
- Tingling and numbness in the forearm, wrist and hand.
- Pain and stiffness interferes with activities of daily living.
- Both elbow joints may be affected.

Home remedies for elbow joint arthritis:
- Excess & repetitive activities of elbow should be reduced.
- OTC pain relievers: Ibuprofen, Naproxen, Acetaminophen.

- Never stop movement of the joint. Keep the joint active. Gentle exercises for the elbow joint is continued.
- Elevation of the elbow if joint swelling is present.
- Healthy and balanced diet.chart
- Anti-inflammatory foods. chart

When to seek medical advice:

- Severe pain and swelling around the elbow.
- Pain on pressure over the joint.
- Pain is accompanied by *fever.*
- Home remedies donot relieve pain.
- Pain interferes the activities of daily life.
- Obvious deformity of the elbow.
- Pain following trauma to the elbow.

Septic arthritis of elbow.

Septic arthritis occurs due to *infection* in the joint. Infants and older age group peoples are mainly affected. The germs travel to the joint through the blood stream from a septic area in the distant part of the body such as skin infection, dental infection, urinary tract infection etc. Septic arthritis may also occur by a penetrating injury which delivers germs directly into the joint. Septic arthritis can quickly and severely damage the cartilage and bone within the joint.

Features of septic arthritis:

- Deep and poorly localised pain within the elbow.
- Swelling of the elbow.
- Fever.
- Overlying skin is red and warm.
- Extreme discomfort and difficulty in using the elbow.

Septic arthritis is a *medical emergency.* It can lead to serious sequele. Therefore prompt recognition and treatment are crucial to ensure a good prognosis.

Pregnancy and Body Pain

Life's biggest miracle is the gift of having life growing inside of you.

Pregnancy is not a disease.

Pregnancy period is a very beautiful and precious time in women life. In this period, a baby grows within the uterus. Pregnancy period extends for about 40 weeks.

Pregnancy almost always is associated with body aches and pains. Some of these discomforts will go away as pregnancy progresses. Some of the aches and pains can easily be managed and prevented by simple home remedies. Rarely medical advices are required.

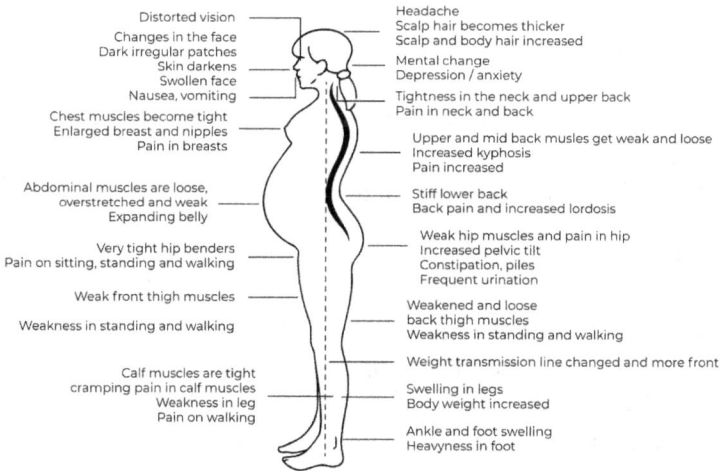

Changes in the body during pregnancy

© Dr. Abu Hena Mahboob

BODY PAIN AND PAIN RELIEF

Changes in the skeleton during pregnancy:

- Reduction of calcium of bones (osteoporosis).
- Loosening of joints due to softening of ligaments by relaxing hormones. Loosening mostly seen in the hip area.
- Relaxed muscles and ligaments causing less strength in movements and increases the risk of falls.
- Changes in spinal curvature causing re-distribution of body weights and changes of stress points. All these predisposes to back pain.
- Changes in gait pattern causes back pain and risk of falls.
- Weight gain.

Body pains in pregnancy.

Pregnancy induced hormonal and physical changes increase the risk of body pains in pregnancy. Stress on the spine, pelvis and genital parts may lead to the following pains:

- Non-specific body pain.
- Lower abdominal pain and cramps.
- Aches and pains in the *back, abdomen, groin and thighs*.
- Back pain with or without radiation to one or both legs.
- Pain in the hip area due to the pressure of the baby's head, increased weight and loosening of joints. Pain can occur at the front or back of the pelvis, sometimes with radiation to the legs. The pain can be achy, sharp, radiating or burning.
- Pain due to *nerve compression*.
- Joint pain due to lax ligaments causing loosening of joints.
- Sharp pain due to cramping of expanding *uterus*.
- Pain due to stretching of the genital organs. These are sharp pain in the lower abdomen on either or both sides.

Other pains.

- Pain abdomen due to *constipation, gas and bloating*.
- *Headache. Heart burn* and indigestion.
- Swollen and tender *breasts*.
- *Dental* pain and sensitivity.
- *Varicose* (dilatation of veins) veins and hemorrhoids (dilated veins in the anus).

Back pain during pregnancy

Back pain during pregnancy is a very common complaint, especially in the early stages. Though the pain is not surprising, but it still deserves proper attention. About 50-80% of pregnant women suffer. Pain can range from mild pain associated with specific activities to acute pain that may become chronic. About 10% of the time the pain becomes so severe that it can interfere with the ability to work or carry out normal activities.

Back pain usually occurs between the 5th and 7th months of pregnancy. In some cases it begins as early as in 2nd month. Women with pre-existing lower back problems are at higher risk for back pains and pain can start at an earlier period.

Causes of back pain during pregnancy:
- Rapid *weight gain*.
- Rapid *postural* changes.
- Changes in the center of gravity of the body.
- Previous *history* of back pain.
- Repetitive *lifting of weights* and *bending forwards*.
- *Pelvic insufficiency*, it is the limited mobility due to low back pain or pelvic pain. These occur due to hormonal changes.
- *Vascular effects*, dilatations of blood vessels.

Home remedies and prevention of back pain and pelvic pains:

It is very common to get back pain or low back pain during pregnancy, especially in the early pregnancy. During pregnancy, the ligaments in the body naturally becomes softer, relaxed and stretched and prepares the pelvis and birth canal for labour. Strain on the joints of lower back and pelvis will cause back pain. Following home remedies may be beneficial:
- Staying *active* is beneficial. *'Motion is lotion'* in back pain. Walk atleast one minute in every hour.
- Maintenance of good posture:
  o Comfortably *wide stance* is maintained during standing.
  o For *standing* long period of time, one foot should rest on a low step stool alternatively.
  o For sitting, back should be kept straight, a chair should be chosen that support the back. Cushion of the chair should be firm, not soft. A small firm pillow or a *maternity support pillow* may be placed behind the lower back.

- - Body should be kept straight during standing with wide stance. Knees should not be locked, that is knees should not be tightly straightened. Keeping slight bending of the knees is better.
  - Chest should be held high. Shoulder relaxed.
- Wearing of *low-heeled* shoes. High heel and flat shoes should be avoided. Sometimes a good arch support for feet gives better result.
- *Maternity support belt* may be used.
- Lifting of weight should be avoided. Self ability and limitations should always be in mind. For lifting a small object, squat down near the object is needed and lifting done with straightening the knees and hips. Back should be kept straight. Bending at the waist and lifting with tension on the back must be avoided.
- *Firm bed* should be used for sleeping. Back pain can make it difficult to find a comfortable sleeping position.
- Never to sleep on the back. Sleeping on one side or the other is recommended. Both knees should be kept bent with a support pillow between the bent knees. Pregnancy pillow may be used under the abdomen and behind back.
- Application of a *heating pad* or *ice pack* to the back may help to some extent.
- *Massage* to the back muscles may also help by improving blood supply to the area.
- Regular *physical activities* are adviced. Physical activities will keep the back strong and may relieve pain.
- *Low-impact exercises* are adviced. Walking and water exercises are beneficial. *Stretching exercises* for the back muscles are also helpful. A trained physiotherapist may help.
- Exercises like squats, lunges, buttock kickbacks, or bridges strengthens buttock muscles, back, thigh muscles and calves and will help to prevent back pain.
- Deep breathing exercises are adviced. chart
- Pelvic floor physiotherapy.
  - *Kegels exercise.* Kegel exercises help to strengthen the pelvic floor muscles.
  - *Squats. Bridge. Bird Dog exercise.* see You tube video.
- *Meditation* for mindfullness.
- Pre-natal *yoga*. Enough sleep. Warm bath.
- Twisting of the body and spine should be avoided by moving the feet when to turn.

- Paracetamol may be taken to ease back pain unless physicians or midwife says not to take.

When to seek medical advice:

- Severe back pain which persists for more than 2 weeks.
- Cramps at regular intervals and gradually intensify.
- Back pain is associated with the following conditions:
    o Second or third trimester.
    o Fever.
    o Bleeding through vagina or pain during micturation.
    o Pain in one or more of sides of the body under ribs.

Heartburn and indigestion

There are some pregnancy hormones which cause relaxation of the valve between the food tube (esophagus) and stomach. Stomach contents are highly acidic. This acidic content may leakback into the esophagus due to relaxation of the valve and causes heartburn.

Home remedies and prevention:

- Avoid lying down just after a meal, ideally for 2 hours.
- Dinner should be earlier in the evening and never just before bed.
- It is most effective if small but frequent meals are taken.
- Eat slowly and chew every bite thoroughly.
- A before-bed light food is better.
- Wear loose cloth in bed.
- Quit smoking.
- Elevation of the headside of bed with a wedge. Pillows alone won't be as effective.
- Pregnancy weight gain should be gradual and moderate.
- *Mind relaxation* by prenatal Yoga and meditation.
- *Avoidence* of certain foods and food habits that can trigger heartburn. They are:
    o Taking of food and drinks at the same time. It is better to take drink atleast 1 hour after a meal.
    o Fried and spicy foods. Fatty foods. Chocolate.
    o Caffeine. Processed meat. Citrus fruits.
    o Carbonated drinks. Mint drinks.
- OTC drugs: Antacids, Omeprazoles, Ranitidines.

When to seek medical advice:

- Heartburn with associated stomach pain.
- Home remedies can't control heartburn.
- Difficulty in eating or keeping food down.
- Unexplained weight loss.
- Loss of appetite.

Feet and ankles swelling

Growing uterus with the baby inside gives pressure over the blood vessels in the pelvis and retards flow of blood to the heart from the lower limbs. Some hormones of pregnancy also acts to retain more fluid in the body. Combination of all these effects will cause increased pressure in the pelvic and lower limb vessels. Increased pressure forces fluid to leave the blood vessels and move into the surrounding tissues and causes swelling in the feet and ankles. This is seen during the later months of pregnancy and this type of swelling goes away spontaneously after giving birth to the baby.

Home remedies and prevention:

- During sitting posture, the feet and ankles should be kept elevated above the level of the seat.
- Waist-high compression stocking wear is helpfull.
- Foot end of the bed may be kept elevated to 3-4 inches.
- Sleeping on left lateral side is more beneficial than on right lateral side.
- Must remain physically active. Atleast one minute of walking in every hour is adviced.
- It is better to wear loose clothing.
- Walking in a pool will compress tissues in the legs and feet and reduce swelling.
- Foods to avoid:
  o Extra salt. Salty foods, sauces and canned foods.
  o Fast foods of backary. Refined sugar.
- Foods to take:
  o Lean protein like fish, poultry, white of egg.
  o Whole grains.
  o Potassium rich foods: chart.

When to seek medical advice:

- To exclude preeclampsia.
- Home remedies do not improve the condition.

Lower abdominal cramps

Lower abdominal cramping pain may be experienced during pregnancy. It may occur in the first month or on the later periods of pregnancy.

At about 2 weeks following conception, light cramping accompanied by scanty vaginal bleeding may occur. This is known as *'implantation bleeding'*. Sometimes a sharp pain or muscle cramp is present in the lower abdomen. At the end of second trimester and into the third a stronger muscle cramp may be experienced which increases in intensity as the date of labour approaches.

This type of pain is relieved by taking rest and low-impact exercises like walking and swimming. Rarely advice from midwives may be needed.

Home remedies for lower abdominal *cramps:*

There are many causes of abdominal cramp during pregnancy. Pregnancy cramp relief depends on the cause of pain. The following home remedies can relieve the most common causes of abdominal cramps during pregnancy.

- *Proper hydration* of the body is beneficial. Plenty of water drinking may ease any cramping related to dehydration, bloating or constipation.
- *Warm bath* (not hot bath) is helpful. Warm bath can help to ease pregnancy cramps related to increased uterine blood flow.
- Body and mind *relaxation* by taking rest in bed. Lying down in bed can relieve pregnancy cramps related to implantation, orgasm, increased blood flow to the uterus and uterine ligament pain. Bed should be firm. Left lateral lying posture with knees bent and a *support pillow* for the abdomen and back gives added benefits.
- Use of *maternity support belt* and *maternity pillow* can help to relieve abdominal cramps linked to uterine ligament stretching pain in the second half of pregnancy.
- Change of posture. Standing to lying down and side changes for lying may be beneficial.

BODY PAIN AND PAIN RELIEF

When to seek medical advice:

Severe lower abdominal cramp and pain that doesn't subside by home remedies.

- Severe lower abdominal pain and cramp accompanied by vaginal bleeding.
- A sudden increase in thirst and a decrease in urination.
- Sudden severe headache accompanied by:
  - Vision changes.
  - Unexplained excess weight gain.
  - Sudden ankle swelling.
  - Abnormally high blood pressure.

These are features of *pre-eclampsia*.

- High fever and or chills.
- Heavy vaginal bleeding and lower abdominal cramp.
- Bloody diarrhea.
- Pain or burning during micturation. Difficulty in micturation or blood in urine.
- Dizziness or feeling of fainting.

Headaches

During pregnancy, some hormone secretion increases many folds. These hormones may trigger headache. Following home remedies may help:

- Meditation and relaxation tactice.
- Headache triggers, like food or odors should be avoided.
- Enough sleep. Cool compression in head.
- Low-impact exercises, e.g,
  - brisk walking, it does not strain joints and muscles.
  - Swimming. Riding a stationary bike.
  - Yoga.
- Jogging and jumping should be avoided.
- Mental stress must be relieved.
- Healthy and balanced diet.chart.

When to seek medical advice:

- Sudden, severe and persistent headache.
- Headache is accompanied by fainting, dizziness and blurred vision. Headache with features of preeclampsia.

Swollen and tender breasts

This is seen in the first trimester. Hormone changes are responsible to make breasts feel sore, sensitive and swollen. These discomforts will subside after few weeks when body has adjusted to the new hormone environments.

Home remedies:

- Wearing a firm support bra is beneficial. The bra should be larger that won't squish the breasts.
- A sports bra may be used during exercise.
- OTC pain relievers. Must consult with your midwife.
- Heat or cold compression in breast.
- Avoid caffeine. Salt intake should be reduced.
- Low fat and high fiber diet is better.
- Vitamin B_6 and Vitamin E supplementation.
- Meditation and mindfullness. Relieve of anxiety.

Feeling of heavyness and pain in the lower abdomen

As the baby grows, the uterus also grows gradually. The weight of the uterus with the baby inside stretches the tissues which suspends the uterus with the pelvic wall and causes pain. It is a kind of *'growing pain'*. As the baby grows, the stretching and pain increases.

Home remedies and prevention:

- Movements like standing and walking hould be slower.
- Never to rise too quickly from sitting or lying position.
- Sudden movements are strictly avoided.
- Warm bath (not hot bath). Swimming in a warm pool.
- Use of maternity belt, maternity pillow and abdominal support garments are beneficial.

Varicose veins and hemorrhoids

Varicose veins are dilated veins and develop in some women during pregnancy. Varicose veins develop in valva, around the anus and lower rectum. Varicose veins in pregnancy is predisposed by the following factors:

- Increased blood volume in the body.
- Decreased return of blood from the lower limb due to pressure of the baby's head in the pelvic veins.
- Hormonal effects.

BODY PAIN AND PAIN RELIEF

Home remedies and prevention:

- To be seated in a chair with the feet placing up above the seat level. This should be practiced whenever get chance.
- Long term standing should be avoided.
- Pregnancy body weight should be monitored regularly. Increase in body weight will increase the chance of varicose vein formation.
- Use of support hose for foot, ankle and leg.
- High fiber and balanced diet.chart
- Extra salt in diet should be avoided.
- Plenty of water intake.
- Constipation must be strictly controlled.

When to seek medical advice:

- To exclude preeclampsia.
- To exclude pregnancy outside uterus cavity.
- Severe abdominal or pelvic pain and vaginal bleeding.

Dental pain

Dental pain and sensitivity is mostly seen at around the second trimester. Gums may feel more sensitive while flossing and brushing. Sometimes gums even bleed. Pregnancy related inflammation of the gum is the main cause. Inflammation may cause swelling of the gum, redness and bleeding during brushing. Loosening of teeth is also seen, which is due to vomiting in the early pregnancy. The acid of vomit causes this effect.

Home remedies and prevention:

- Brushing with a soft brush and flossing.
- Rinsing with salt water is beneficial.
- Softer tooth brush use.
- Good oral hygiene should be maintained.

When to seek medical advice:

- Severe symptoms and not responding to home remedies.
- Gum is painful on touching and brushing.
- Gum infection is suspected.
- Foul smell in the mouth.

Pregnancy and Body Pain

Pregnancy symptoms which must not be ignored:

- Extreme vomiting. Vaginal bleeding.
- Severe headache. Intense abdominal pain. High fever.
- Lots of watery vaginal discharge. Painful urination.
- Itching all over the body.
- Lack of fetal movement.
- Pain in the calf muscle.

Rheumatoid Arthritis (RA)

Giving up is not an option.

Rheumatoid arthritis (RA) is one of the most common causes of joint pain. It is a long term inflammatory joint disease. Rheumatoid arthritis is an autoimmune disease.

The immune system in the body normally makes specialized cells and chemicals called antibodies, that attack bacteria, viruses and other organisms and abnormal cells. Thus, it helps to fight against infection and other diseases.

Autoimmune disease is a misdirected immune response that occurs when the immune system goes awry and attacks the cells of self body. Here, the immune system of the body attacks the healthy body cells and causes inflammation and tissue destruction.

Rheumatoid arthritis occurs when the immune system of the body sends antibodies mistakenly against it's own. The antibodies act against the lining of synovial joints called the synovial membrane, synovial coverings of tendons and ligaments etc.

The synovial membrane is the inner lining of the capsule that surrounds the joints. The resulting inflammation thickens the synovium and releases some chemicals which ultimately can destroy the nearby cartilage, bone, ligaments and tendons associated with the joint.

Tendons and ligaments that hold the joint together becomes weaker by rheumatoid arthritis. Gradually, the joint loses its shape and alignment. Destruction of cartilage covering of bones occur. Inflammation and destruction of structures ultimately results in osteoarthritis.

Causes of rheumatoid arthritis:

- Exact cause is not known.
- There are some *risk factors* which may predispose to the development of RA.

Risk factors for RA:

There are several factors that may increase the risk of developing RA. They are:

- *Female sex:* Estrogen hormone may be responsible.
- *Age:* RA can occur at any age, most common in the middle age group (30-60 yrs).
- *Family history:* RA can run in families. Daughter of an affected mother with RA is 3 times more susceptible.
- Low vitamin D intake.
- *Environmental exposure:* Air pollution, exposure to silica, dust, asbestos, tobacco smoke and other smokes.
- *Obesity:* Obese females are at a higher risk of developing RA.
- *Infection:* Teeth infection, any long term bacterial and some viral infections in the body.
- Repeated exposure to extreme heat or cold.
- Mental stress, anxiety. Major trauma to the body.
- *Diet:* Red meat, fatty foods, Processed foods. High salt intake.
- Contact with pesticides, diesel, petrol, kerosine.
- Lower socio-economic group of people.

Which organs are mainly affected in RA?

- Most joints in the body.
- Muscles which are attached to any bone.
- Lungs, eyes, skin, heart.
- Blood vessels: causes inflammation of blood vessels and reduces blood supply to different organs.
- Spleen: Involvement of spleen will increase the susceptibility to infection.

RA can affect any synovial joint in the body. At the begining, the small joints of the hands and feet are affected. Both sides of the body are usually affected at the same time, in the same way. But these does not always happen.

Small fleshy lumps, called rheumatoid nodules may form under the skin around the affected joints. These nodules may be painful.

Rheumatoid Arthritis (RA)

Early symptoms of RA:

- Feeling of weakness and fatigue.
- Low grade fever. Feeling of discomfort.
- Unexplained sudden weight loss.
- Morning stiffness in hands and feet.
- Pain in joints.

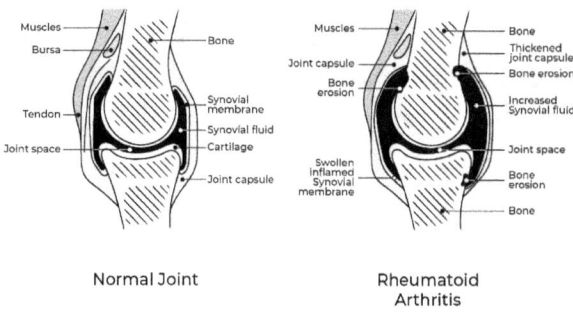

Normal Joint   Rheumatoid Arthritis

Features of RA.

The main features of RA are:

- Joint pain. Joint swelling, warmth and redness.
- Pain on pressing the joint.
- Joint stiffness, especially in the morning or after a period of inactivity. Stiffness persists for 1-2 hours.
- Range of movement of joint is gradually reduced.
- Gradually, the shape of joints is deformed.
- Tiredness and lack of energy.
- Poor appetite and weight loss. Fever, sweating.
- Respiratory distress from involvement of lungs.
- Pain all over the body. Sleep disturbance.
- Anaemia. Depression. Dry eyes. Chest pain.
- Disinterest to the surroundings.

How RA is diagnosed?

There is no single laboratory test to confirm early RA. RA is diagnosed clinically by careful clinical history taking from the patient and also careful clinical examination.

X-rays of the affected joints may show some changes which are related to RA.

Treatment options for RA:

There is no cure for rheumatoid arthritis. Patient may remain relatively symptom free by practicing some advices, taking some medicines and physiotherapy.

Aims of treatment:

- To reduce pain and inflammation.
- To keep the joints supple and active.
- To prevent destruction and deformity of joints.
- To enjoy symptom free life.

Prevention of rheumatoid arthritis:

There is no definite known cause of RA. So, there is no definite way of prevention. There are some predisposing or risk factors which are although non-specific, even than can be avoided and lower the chances of the disease.

- Maintenance of healthy body weight.chart
- Smoking and Alcohol consumption reduced.
- Control of diabetes.
- Avoidence of polluted environment.
- Chronic infection in the body should be timely treated.
- Stress and anxiety avoided. Relaxed life style is beneficial.
- Healthy and balanced diet.chart.
- Foods causing inflammation avoided.chart
- Avoidence of injury to the body. Repeated pushing, pulling or lifting of heavy objects must be avoided.
- Regular physical exercise and stretching. Swimming, cycling, yoga can delay the complications of RA.
- Treatment of RA should be started early. It will make symptoms less painful and save the joints from damage.

Home remedies for rheumatoid arthritis:

- Healthy and balanced *diet*.
- Maintenance of healthy *body weight*.
- Getting enough *sleep*, atleast 8 hours of sleep every night. Taking a nap during the afternoon may also help.
- Regular *physical exercise* is important to strengthen muscles and increase joint range of movement. Low-impact exercises like brisk walking, swimming and warm water aerobics are usually good.
- *Yoga*. Yoga offers individualized exercises along with potential benefits from breathing and meditation. Yoga improves mood and acceptance of fatigue and chronic pain in younger people. Yoga may also reduce pain and inflammation, improves joint flexibility and function and lower stress and tension for better sleep and improves quality of life.
- *Meditation* has been used to help focus the mind and soothe the spirit. Here meditation is done by focusing on breathing and just noticing each inhale and exhale and it is beneficial. Meditation is good for soul and reduces the inflammation response caused by stress. Meditation reduces stress, controls anxiety, improves sleep, helps to control pain, promotes emotional health, enhances self-awareness and help to ease pain caused by all types of arthritis.
- *Massage*. Moderate pressure massage can improve healthy circulation throughout the arthritic joints. First sore points in the body are identified and moderate pressure massage is applied. It reduces pain and swelling and helps to improve joint function, increases grip strength and increases range of motion of joints. Sleep quality and daytime energy levels are improved and ultimately improves quality of life. Massage should be avoided on affected joints during flare up of inflammation.
- *Tai chi*. Tai chi combines deep breathing and relaxation with slow and gentle movements. Tai chi is very calming and peaceful. Tai chi exercises the mind, body and spirit. It may reduce anxiety, stress, improves balance and physical function and arthritis pain relief. Tai chi can cause significant improvement in the range of motion of the joints of the lower extremity in the older people. Tai chi may cause higher levels of participation in exercise programme and enjoyment of exercises.
- *Heat and cold compression* is beneficial to inflamed joints. Cold compression checks joint swelling and inflammation. Heat compression relaxes muscles and increases blood flow. Moist heating pad or a warm, dump towel may be used. Getting too hot should be avoided. Warm

water shower is beneficial. Hot tub bath may also be used. It relaxes stiff muscles.
- OTC pain relievers: Ibuprofen, Naproxen, Piroxicum.
- Creams, gels and lotions are available for topical use. They can be rubbed directly onto the skin to help to ease painful joints.
- Assistive devices like *splints* and *braces* stabilize and give rest to the inflamed joints. They reduce pain and swelling. They improve grip strength and skill of limbs.
- *Support from the family,* friends and clubs improves quality of life. Patients become confident in managing the symptoms.

Foods and Rheumatoid arthritis

Foods those must be *avoided:*

These foods can trigger the body to produce pro-inflammatory chemicals and increase inflammation.see chart

Some vegetables are *bad* for arthritis. They contain solanine and is responsible for aggravation of inflammation and pain. They are: Eggplants. Peppers. Tomatoes, etc.

Foods beneficial to Rheumatoid arthritis (anti-inflammatory foods). chart

Herbs and spices:
- *Ginger:* It is anti-inflammatory.
- *Green* tea: contains polyphenols which acts as anti-oxident.
- *Turmeric:* contains curcumin.It is anti-inflammatory.
- *Cinnamon:* It is an anti-oxident and inhibits cell damage.
- *Garlic:* contains diallyl disulfide. It is an anti-inflammatory chemical.
- *Black peeper:* It is an anti-oxident, anti-microbial, anti-inflammatory and gastro-protective agent.
- *Willow bark:* It is anti-inflammatory agent.
- *Indian frankincense extract.* It has many properties:
  o Anti-inflammtory and analgesic effects.
  o Inhibit autoimmune process.
  o Prevent cartilage loss.
- *Borage seed oil:* Improves joint tenderness, swelling and joint pain.
- *Devil's claw:*
  o Anti-inflammatory.

- o Improves joint pain, stiffness and joint function in the hand, wrist, elbow, shoulder, hip, knee and back.
- *Thunder god vine:*
  - o Anti-inflammatory.
  - o Changes the immune system.
  - o Relieves pain and inflammation in rheumatoid arthritis.
- *Green-lipped Mussel extract.*
  - o Anti-inflammatory.
  - o Joint-protecting properties.

Best fruits for Rheumatoid arthritis:

- Fruits with dark red colour: they have flavonoid anthocyanin, ascorbic acid (vitamin C) and carotenoids. They have powerful anti-inflammatory and anti oxidant properties. Some flavonoid rich foods are:
  - o All berries, Red cabbage, kale, lettuce.
  - o Green tea. Dark chocolates. onion.
  - o Red grapes, red wine, Peaches, Parsley.
- Citrus fruits, Cherries.
- Strawberries, red raspberries: They are naturally low sugar and have more vitamin C. They control high blood pressure and cholesterol.
- Avocado: contains anti-inflammatory mono-unsaturated fat, vitamin E.
- Water melon reduces CRP. It is high in beta-cryptoxanthin and reduce the risk of RA.
- Grapes contain resveratrol and other beneficial anti-oxidents and other polyphenols.

Omega-3 fatty acid rich foods. see chart

When to seek medical advice:

- Pain, swelling and stiffness in fingers and toes.
- Fever and respiratory distress. Chest pain.
- Malaise, weakness, fatigue, tiredness.
- Symptoms present on both sides of the body.
- On giving pressure over the joint if it feels pain.

Shoulder Pain

We all need a shoulder to cry on

—Anonymous

The joint at the upper part of the arm is the shoulder joint. The part of the body from shoulder joint to root of the neck is the shoulder. The shoulder joint is the main joint of the shoulder.

The shoulder joint must be mobile enough for the wide range of actions of the arm and the hand. The joint is also stable enough to allow for actions such as lifting heavy weights, pushing and pulling.

Shoulder joint allows 360^0 of rotational movement to the arm. The joint allows the arm to hinge out and up away from the body. Shoulder joint disorders are the most common causes of shoulder pain.

The shoulder is made up of three bones and associated muscles, ligaments, tendons, nerves and blood vessels.

The bones are:

- Collar bone (the clavicle).
- Shoulder blade (the scapula), and
- Upper arm bone (the humerus).

We hang bags (back-pack), carry weight over the shoulder and over-stretch the shoulder joint during different activities. These activities cause pain in the shoulder.

Shoulder pain is special for some reasons. Many pains in the shoulder region are due to causes related to the shoulder structures like shoulder joint and bones, muscles, ligaments, tendons, nerves and blood vessels of shoulder and shoulder joint. Other pains of shoulder region originate in a distant structures and are referred to the shoulder area. These pains are called *referred shoulder pain*.

Causes of *referred* shoulder pain:

- *Pain from the heart:* pain is felt in the chest, back, neck, jaw, left arm, shoulder and in many other places.
- *Gallbladder pain:* pain referred to right shoulder.
- *Pain from pancreas:* is referred to shoulder and back.
- *Pains from the lungs and bronchus:* pneumonia, cancer.
- *Ovarian tumour pain* may come to the shoulder.
- *Pain from the liver* diseases: referred to right shoulder.

When to suspect a referred pain?

Referred shoulder pain is felt in the shoulder but no pain felt on moving the shoulder joint. Referred shoulder pain may be associated with any of the following symptoms:

- Chest pain. Respiratory distress.
- Irregular pulse rate.
- Sudden profuse sweating. Light headedness.
- Blood in the sputum. Fever.
- Difficulty in vision. Weakness in the limbs.
- Loss of consciousness.

Many of the conditions mentioned above are of medical and surgical emergencies. Patient should be immediately shifted to the hospital.

Shoulder joint pain

The shoulder joint comprises the part of the body where the upper end of the arm bone forms joint to the shoulder blade, the scapula. Shoulder joint is a major joint of the shoulder. It also includes another joint called acromioclavicular joint which is formed by collar bone and shoulder blade (scapula).

Shoulder joint is one of the most mobile joint in the body. It can move in all directions, above-below, front-back and in circular directions. This mobility provides the upper extremity with tremendous range of motion. *'Rotator cuff'* is responsible for this wide range of motion. *'Rotator cuff'* is formed by four tendons and is intimately adjacent to the joint capsule. *'Rotator cuff'* may be affected by infection, inflammation and other conditions of the joint and cause pain.

Causes of shoulder joint pain:

- Injury and inflammation of any tissue directly related to shoulder. Injury or torn of any cartilage.
- Injury causing torn, sprain or strain to rotator cuff.
- Rupture of any tendon around the shoulder joint.
- Inflammed bursa around the shoulder.
- Inflammation of any tendon (tendonitis) related to the shoulder. Bone and joint infection.
- Pinched nerve in the neck or shoulder (cervical radiculopathy).
- Broken bone in and around shoulder.
- Frozen shoulder.
- Tumour of any structure in the shoulder region.
- Calcific inflammation of tendons.
- Dislocation of any joint in the shoulder area.
- Rheumatoid arthritis and osteoarthritis.
- Avascular necrosis of any bone.
- Nerve injury.
- Injury to any structure which enter the chest cavity from neck region.

When to seek emergency treatment?

- Shoulder joint pain following a trauma.
- Dislocation of any joint of shoulder region.
- Shoulder pain associated with fever and stiffness of neck.
- Deformed shoulder joint and adjacent area.
- Sudden swelling of the shoulder.
- Sudden severe pain in the shoulder area and inability to move the joint.

Home treatment for shoulder joint pain:

- Completely stopping the use of shoulder joint is not recommended. Some movements of shoulder joint must be continued. One minute of movement in every hour may be done.
- Rest for few days in an elbow bag.
- OTC pain relievers: Ibuprofen. Naproxen. Acetaminophen.
- Cold compress: can reduce swelling in the shoulder.
- Heating pad use.

BODY PAIN AND PAIN RELIEF

- Rolling shoulders up and back against a wall and then letting them to relax down is beneficial. It will prevent rounded shoulder posture which is unhealthy.
- Slowly return to regular activities and activity modification.

Prevention of shoulder joint pain:

- If any work or movement hurts the shoulder, it should be avoided.
- Completely stopping the use of shoulder is not beneficial. This can make the pain worse.
- Use of good posture for sitting, standing, walking or any physical work. Slouch during sitting should be avoided.
- Sitting and standing should be with straight back and with the shoulders down and gently back.
- If pain is severe, sitting with a cushion on the lap to support the arm is beneficial.
- It is better to avoid rounded shoulder posture or, bringing the neck forward. Standing against a wall and making contact with hips, upper back and head can stretch and make a good posture for shoulder.
- Safe weight lifting rules must be followed.
- Take a break for a couple of minutes every hour during work. Move around and stretching is good.
- For desk work, the set-up should be such that it is comfortably used. Strain in the neck must be avoided.
- Do not strain to reach what you want. Step stool must be used to reach high places.
- Body should be kept in good physical shape with regular exercise and stretching.
- Healthy and balanced diet.chart
- Strenuous exercise should be avoided. Poor exercise technique can cause additional damage and create more trouble.
- Must warm-up before starting any heavy physical activity.
- Increasing strength and flexibility of the shoulder are the best way to keep the shoulders healthy and prevent injuries.

When to seek medical advice:

- Shoulder pain with no obvious injury.
- Pain in the shoulder even when not using the arm.
- Shoulder pain is accompanied by:
  - Fever. Swelling of the joint.

- o   Redness in the skin over the shoulder.
- o   Tenderness and warmth around the joint.
- o   Arm numbness, weakness or paralysis.
- Intense pain in the joint.
- Sudden swelling of the joint.
- Persistent shoulder pain that has lasted for longer than a week or cannot be relieved by home treatments.
- Unstable shoulder joint.
- Shoulder pain causing sleep disturbances.
- Difficulty or pain when attempting to reach backwards, to raise the arm over the head or to reach accross the body.
- An apparent abnormality or deformity of the shoulder.
- A snapping, clicking or popping sound in the shoulder, particularly when lifting or throwing.
- New swelling or a lump around the shoulder.

Wrist Pain

'The world is like a broken wrist that healed the wrong way, and will never be the same again'

—F. Hardinge

The wrist is a complex joint that bridges the hand to the forearm. Wrist joint is a biaxial joint and can bend forward and backward. In order to maintain mobility without sacrificing stability, the wrist joint has a complex configuration of ligaments and shapes of bones.

The wrist region includes the carpal tunnel, the anatomical snuff-box, bracelet lines and the deep tough tissues covering on the front and back of wrist.

There are 8 bones and more than 30 muscles control the hand and wrist movements. These muscles are in the hand, wrist and forearms. Muscles are attached to bones by tendons. The innermost covering of joint is a special type of membrane called synovial membrane. Wrist joint is a synovial joint.

Tendons are multiple strong bands of tissue that cross over the wrist. Tendons connect the muscles in the forearm to the hand and finger bones. Tendons located on the palm side of the hand allow fingers to bend for grasping and gripping objects. Tendons on the top side of the hand help the fingers to straighten and release of grapsed objects.

Ligaments are short bands of tough, flexible tissue. Ligaments connect two bones together, particularly in the joints. Ligaments are like strong, firmly attached strapes or ropes. They stabilize the joint or hold the ends of two bones together. Ligaments ensure that the bones in the joint donot twist too much or move too far apart and become dislocated.

Most cases of hand and wrist pain will not be a sign of a serious or long-term problem. They will settle in a few days or weeks with some simple self-care at home.

Causes of *wrist pain:*

- *Trauma* to the wrist:
    - Sprain. Strain. Broken bones.
    - Blow or fall on the wrist.
    - Overuse injury to the wrist.
- *Inflammation:*
    - Joint: Arthritis, like rheumatoid arthritis, Osteoarthritis and other rare form of arthritis.
    - Tendon: Tendonitis, Tenosynovitis (de Quervain's tenosynovitis).
    - Capsule of joint: Capsulitis.
- *Infection:*
    - Osteomyelitis of bones of wrist joint.
    - Septic arthritis of the joint.
    - Infection of other soft tissues.
- *Pressure to the nerve:*
    - Median nerve (Carpal Tunnel syndrome).
    - Ulnar nerve.
- *Osteoporosis* and broken bones:
    - Scaphoid fracture.
    - Colles' fracture.
- *Tumor* of any component of wrist:
    - Bone tumour.
    - Tumours of synovial membrane.
    - Tumours of tendon, ganglion cyst.

Symptoms that may occur along with wrist pain:

Depending on the cause, symptoms may be mild at the start. Symptoms may become worse as time goes on. Wrist pain may be accompanied by the following symptoms:

- *Swelling* of the wrist, hand and fingers.
- *Stiffness* of the wrist and difficulties in making a fist or grip.
- *Swelling, redness* and *warmth* around the wrist.
- Fever.
- Sudden sharp pain in the hand.

- Feeling of prickling and numbness in the hand and fingers.
- Pain, *numbness* or prickling gets worse at night.
- A *clicking sound* when moving the wrist.

Identifying different types of wrist pain.

Wrist sprain

Wrist sprain occurs when the ligaments of the wrist are stretched beyond their normal limits. This occurs after an injury such as fall onto the ground, punch or blow with the fist.

Features of wrist sprain:

- *Pain* at rest and also with the movement of the wrist.
- *Swelling* around the wrist.
- *Bruising* or *discoloration* of the overlying skin.
- *Burning* or *tingling* sensations in the wrist and hand.

Inflammation of wrist tendons (tendonitis)

Several tendons cross the wrist. When one or more tendons are inflamed, wrist tendonitis develops. Occupational and sports activities that involve repetitive wrist motion, such as use of keyboard, working with machinary and sports that cause repetitive stress on the wrist like tennis, badminton, boxing, golf are the common causes of wrist tendonitis. Sometimes exact cause may not be known.

Features of *wrist tendonitis:*

- Dull aching pain in the wrist.
- Stiffness of wrist especially in the morning.
- Swelling and warmth in the wrist.
- A popping sensation may be felt in the wrist when moving the joint.

Inflammation of tendon covering (tenosynovitis)

Tendons in the wrist are covered by synovial membrane and forms a tendon sheath. Tendon sheaths are fluid filled synovial covering and allow the tendons to glide as it passes through the wrist tunnel. Inflammation of the tendon sheath is called tenosynovitis. The features are same as tendonitis.

de Quervain's tenosynovitis is a specific type of inflammation of tendon sheath. It causes wrist pain on the thumb side of the wrist. The pain may be felt in the hand and forearm also. This type of tenosynovitis is most common in middle aged women and recurr frequently. Baby care and jobs or hobbies that involve repetitive hand and wrist motion greatly predispose the condition. Important features of de Quervain's disease are:

- Pain and swelling near the base of the thumb.
- Grasping or pinching causes pain.
- A sense of 'sticking' or stop-and-go sensation in moving the thumb.

Carpal Tunnel Syndrome (CTS). see hand pain.

Inflammation of wrist joints (arthritis)

There are a few different types of arthritis that may affect the wrist. They are:

- Rheumatoid arthritis (RA).
- Gout arthritis.
- Osteoarthritis(OA).
- Bacterial (septic) arthritis.

Features of rheumatoid arthritis(RA).see RA

Features of gouty arthritis.see gout and body pain

Features of osteoarthritis(OA):

- Pain in the wrist especially after hand activity.
- Stiffness, tenderness and swelling in the wrist.
- Grating sensation in wrist.
- Bone spur formation in wrist joint bones.

Septic arthritis of wrist

This is due to bacterial infection of wrist joint. Organisms reach the wrist joint by blood borne from a distant infected site or direcly through an open wound and establish an infection.

Features of septic arthritis of wrist:

- Pain,swelling and warmth in the wrist.
- Fever and chills.
- Inability to move the joint.
- Fatigue and generalized weakness.

Wrist fracture

Wrist fracture is common in old age. This may occur due to an injury and/or bone weakness such as with osteoporosis. Common type of wrist fractures are *scaphoid fracture* and *Colles' fracture.*

Features of wrist fracture:

- History of trauma to the wrist.
- Severe pain in wrist that might worsen when gripping or squeezing or moving the hand or wrist.
- Deformity of the wrist, such as a bent wrist.
- Swelling of wrist.
- Pain on touch (tenderness) the wrist.
- Bruising over the skin.

A *scaphoid fracture* may arise from a fall on an outstretched hand. It causes swelling, pain and tenderness in the anatomical snuff-box area. The pain may worsen when a person tries to pinch or grasp something.

Colles' fracture is a type of fracture of the distal forearm in which the broken end of the outer bone of the forearm is bent backwards. Symptoms may include pain, swelling, dinner fork deformity of the wrist and bruising over the skin. The nerve in the wrist canal (median nerve) may be damaged.

Ganglion cyst

These are non-cancerous fluid-filled capsule which develops on a tendon. It sometimes occur on the back of the wrist. They feel smooth and rubbery. Rarely, the cyst may compress a nerve, causing some muscle weakness and or numbness and prickling sensation in the fingers.

Home treatment for *wrist pain:*

- *Avoidence* of tasks that make the pain worse.
- Rest to the wrist. A *splint* for the wrist may be used.
- If swelling is present, *elevation* of the wrist done above the level of the heart/chest.
- OTC pain relievers: acetaminophen, ibuprofen, naproxen.
- Heat and cold *compression*. Heat can loosen stiffness. Cold is effective for hand and wrist pain that results from activity, such as playing Tennis, Badminton, Golf etc.
- Stretching exercises for hand and wrist.

- Compression of wrist by using an elastic bandage. The wrap should be snug, but not cutting off circulation to the hand and wrist (Prickling is a sign that it's too tight).
- Keeping wrist and hand moving. Moving wrist and hand as much as possible can help to ease pain and stiffness. This will also maintain range of movement, function and strength.
- Hydration of the body must be maintained.

When to seek medical advice for wrist pain:

- Pain does not relieve even after 1-2 weeks of home treatment. Pain is getting worse day by day.
- Pain is present even after refraining from activities that caused the pain.
- Pain after trauma to the wrist. Change of shape of wrist after trauma or fall to the ground.
- The pain keeps returning.
- Pain interferes the activities of daily life.
- Pain, swelling, redness, fever or stiffness in the wrist.
- Pain is accompanied by fever over 100^0F.
- Numbness or prickling is becoming worse and there is little or no feeling in the fingers or hand.
- Weakness makes holding things difficult.
- Weakness and a decreased ability to carry out activities such as gripping objects and using a keyboard.
- Simple hand movements are no longer possible.

Prevention of wrist pain:

- Provide rest to the wrist. Avoidence of tasks that make the pain worse.
- Prevention of wrist injury and wearing of protective wrist splints or guards in sports.
- Lifting of heavy objects or grip anything too tightly should be avoided.
- Avoiding repetitive motions and taking breaks between movements.
- Use of proper size and shape mouse and wrist rest in mouse pad.
- Job change may be required in some cases.
- Practice of proper ergonomics.
- Keeping wrist and hand moving. Moving wrist and hand as much as possible can help to ease pain and stiffness. This will also maintain range of movement, function and strength.
- Stretching exercises for wrist:
  o Fist to fan stretch.

- Thumb touches.
- Desk press.
- Range of movement exercises of wrist maintained.
- Use of custom made wide-handled utensils in case of arthritis.
- Use of any jewellery in the wrist region is stopped.

Appendices

Hydration

Hydration is the process of providing an adequate amount of liquid to body tissues. Upto 70% of the human body is water. A normal person with normal kidney can drink as much as *17 litres* of water if taken in slowly without changing their serum sodium level and body function.

Features of less hydration (dehydration)

- Thirst increased. Dry and sticky mouth.
- Not urinating sufficiently. Dark yellow urine.
- Skin feels dry and cool.
- Headache.
- Muscle cramp and pain.

Benefits of proper hydration

- Regulates blood pressure and body temperature.
- Digestion and delivery of nutrients to cells.
- Maintains skin health and beauty.
- Protection of brain and spinal cord.
- Improves sleep quality, cognition and mood.
- Lubricates joints and improves functions.
- Maintains airway.
- Proper kidney function and excretion of wastes.

Proper hydration is mandatory for proper body function.

Healthy body weight

A healthy weight, or normal weight, means that BMI falls within a weight range that is not associated with an increased risk for weight-related diseases and health issuses. Healthy body weight is comfortably maintained with 'normal' healthy eating and regular physical activity.

BMI 18.5 to 24.9 is *normal* or *healthy weight range.*

BODY PAIN AND PAIN RELIEF

Maintenance of healthy body weight.

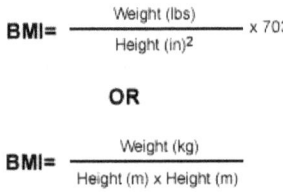

- Limit portion size to control calorie intake. Consultation with a dietician is helpful.
- Never to skip a meal.
- Stay hydrated. Drink sufficient water.
- Be as physically active as can be. Exercise daily.
- Move more and sit less. Walk atleast one minute in every one hour.
- Healthy and balanced diet. chart
- Get sufficient sleep.
- Maintain healthy behavior.
- Physicin consultation about body weight if it is too much or too low.

Benefits of healthy body weight

- Activities of daily life are done more comfortably.
- Body movements are easier.
- Physical exercises are done more effectively.
- Body circulates blood more efficiently.
- Body fluid levels are more easily managed.
- Less chance of development of: heart disease, stroke, high blood pressure, diabetes, certain cancers, gall stones, osteoarthritis, sleep apnea, breathing problems.

Healthy and balanced diet

A balanced diet is a diet that contains different kinds of foods in certain quantities and proportions so that the requirement for calories, proteins, fats, fibres, minerals, vitamins, water is adequate.

Balanced diet should contain:

Fruits and vegetables: 40%.

Protein: 25%.

Fibre rich carbohydrate: 25%.

Fat: 10%.

This should not be a fixed value. It must be individualized. The relative amount should be adjusted after consultation with a dietecian.

- Whole-grain foods: whole wheat bread, oatmeal, brown rice.
- Protein foods: lean meat, fish, poultry without skin, eggs, beans, peas.
- Foods with unsaturated fats (relatively good fat). chart
- Fresh fruits. Dried fruits.
- Green leafy vegetables. chart
- Nuts and seeds. Pulses.
- Fat free and low fat dairy products: Milk, low-fat yogurt, cheeze.
- Soy drinks.

Benefits of balanced diet

- Maintains healthy body weight.
- Strong immune system is maintained.
- Increase energy level of the body.
- Reduce the risk of chronic illness: obesity, diabetes, heart diseases, stroke, cancer, joint diseases.
- Improve mental health, mood, general wellbeing.
- Improve memory and brain health.
- Maintain strong bones and teeth.
- Effects of aging slow down.
- Help to live longer.

High fiber foods

- Boiled peas, lentils, beans.
- Chia seeds. Flax seeds.
- Whole wheat bread, Brown rice, Oatmeal.
- Green leafy vegetables, okra, kale. broccoli.

- Apple with skin. Raw fruits.
- All nuts. Berries.

Green leafy vegetables:

- Kale, Spinach, Cabbage, Broccoli, Brussels sprouts.
- Microgreens, Collard greens, Beet greens, Lettuce.
- Cauliflower, Dandelion greens, Arugula, chard, Bathua.
- Bokchoy, Swiss chard, Watercress, Mustard greens.
- Fenugreek, Moringa.

Vegetables should be raw or moderately cooked.

Microgreen vegetables

Microgreen vegetables are young vegetable greens that are 1-3 inches tall. Microgreens are baby plants and contain more significant amounts of nutrients and health-promoting micronutrients than their mature counterparts.

Common microgreen vegetables are:

- Pea shoots, Radish sprouts, Sunflower shoots, Wheatgrass.
- Cauliflower, Broccoli, Amaranth, Fennel, Muatard, Arugala.
- Beets, Basil, Cabbage, Celery, Chard, Carrot, Onion, Garlic.
- Parsley, leek, Lettuce, Chicory, Cress, Cilanto, Chervil, Sorrel.

Sea vegetables

Sea vegetables are edible seaweed. They grow wild in or near the sea. They are of salty taste. They also grow in the rivers, lakes and other water bodies.

Sea vegetables are packed with protein, iodine, fiber and vitamines A, B, C and E, in amounts that are 10 to 20 times higher than land vegetables. Some sea vegetables contain more calcium than milk. Sea lettuce has 25 times more iron than found in beef.

Common sea vegetables

- Spirulina: contains vitamin E, C, B6. It maintains healthy immune system.
- Kelp: brown algae seaweed.
- Salicornia: sea asparagus, sea bean.
- Dulse: seaweed, rich in iodine.

- Nori: red algae. dried seaweed.
- Kombu: seaweed, reduces cholesterol and controls hypertension.

Foods and inflammation

Foods cause and increase inflammation: (foods to avoid):

- Refined carbohydrates, refined rice and other grains, white breads, pastries. Refined sugar, Added sugar, added salt.
- Saturated fats (bad fats): chart.
- Soda and other sugar-sweetened beverages.
- Processed foods. Artificial chemicals.
- Bakery foods: cookies, candy, ice cream.
- Artificial sweetners, sugar alternatives (Aspartame) and food additives.
- Monosodium glutamate (MSG). This is flavour enhancer in Fast foods, chips, snak foods, seasoning, blends, frozen meals, canned vegetables, soups, processed meats. Condiments. Instant noodle products.
- Red meat, processed meat. Hot dogs, sausages.
- Trans fats in baked goods, cakes, cookies, pies, pastry.
- Canned fruits, Sweetened yogurts.
- Fried foods: french fries, chips, crackers, doughnuts.
- Fast food meals. Excess alcohol.
- Dairy. Non-dairy coffee creamer.
- Margarine. Butter. Lard. Vegetable oils. other unhealthy oils.
- Omega-6 fatty acid containing foods. chart
- Allergic foods which may vary from person to person.

Limit intake of

Gluten.
- Night shades (solanine): tomatoes, eggplants, peppers.

Foods that *reduce inflammation* (beneficial foods).

- Whole cereals and grains. Oatmeals and other high fiber foods. Whole wheat, Brown rice. Chart
- Fatty fish: Salmon, Tuna, Sardins, Mackerel, Herring and other cold water fishes.
- Foods rich in vit.D. Cereals fortified with vit.D, fortified bread, low fat milk fortified with vit.D.
- Fruits: Berries, Cherries, Citrus fruits, Beets, Apple, Bananas, Pomegranates, pine apples.

- All nuts: Almonds, Walnuts, Pistachios.
- Green leafy vegetables: chart
- Un-saturated fats (relatively good fats).chart

Foods with saturated fats (relatively bad fats):
- Full cream milk, white chocolate, toffee.
- Cakes, puddings, cheese. Pastries and pies.
- Processed meat: sausages, burgers, kebabs, bacon.
- Butter, lard, ghee, margarine.
- Cocoanut and palm oils.

Foods with un-saturated fats (relatively good fats)
- Oils from vegetables, seeds and nuts such as: sunflower, safflower, rapeseed, olive, walnut, corn oil, canola oil, pea nuts. Avocado.
- Nuts: almonds, hazel nuts, pecans, walnut etc.
- Seeds: pumpkin, sesame seeds.
- Oily fishes: herring, mackerel, salmon, trout.

Foods with no saturated fat (relatively good fat)
- Fishes high in omega-3: Salmon, Mackerel, Trout, Herring, Sardines,Tuna.
- Lean beef, Lean pork, Lean lamb.
- Skinless chicken or turkey.
- Mushrooms. Olive oils and olives. Avocados.
- Seeds: Flaxseeds, Chia seeds.
- Legumes: lentils.
- Ginger, Turmeric, Garlic, Onion.
- Probiotics and prebiotics. chart
- Green, white and black tea. Coffee not more than one or two cups a day.
- Anti-oxident containing foods. chart
- Omega-3 fatty acid containing foods. chart

Calcium rich foods.
- Milk and dairy products: Cheese. Yogurt.
- Fruits: Fig. Papaya. Oranges. Citrus fruits.
- Fish: Sardins with bones. Salmon. Shrimp. Mackerel.
- Sea foods.
- Dark leafy green vegetables: Collard greens. Kale. Spinach. Turnip greens. Cabbage. Broccoli. Mustard greens. Squash. Arugula. Okra.

- Fortified cereals: Oatmeal. Rice milk. Soymilk. Almond milk. Fortified drinks.
- Seeds: Sesame. Chia seeds. Sunflower seeds. Celery.
- Beans and lentils: All beans. Peas. Legumes. Almond.

Benefits of calcium

- Builds and maintains strong bones and teeth.
- Proper functioning of heart, nerves and muscles.
- Protects against cancer, diabetes and high blood pressure.
- Lowers the risks of eclampsia.
- Calcium is a co-factor for many enzymes.
- Calcium deficiency causes:
    - muscle cramp, spasm and fatigue.
    - Tingling and numbness in hands and feet.
    - irregular heart rhythm.

Iron rich foods

- Red meat. Poultry. Egg. Liver. Fishes. Oyster. Shellfish. Clams. Other sea foods.
- Dark green leafy vegetables. Beet. Peas. Beans. Legumes. Lentils. Soybeans.
- Dried and fresh fruits: Raisin. Dates. Apricots. Apple. Berries. Nuts and seeds.
- Iron fortified foods. Dark chocolate.

Benefits of iron

- Boosts hemoglobin formation. Hemoglobin carries oxygen to body cells. Improves brain and muscle function.
- Maintains growth and development.
- Regulates body temperature, nerve functions.
- Prevents and manage chronic diseases.
- Treatment of anemia and restless leg syndrome.
- Boosts up immunity and general body energy.
- Maintains proper gastrointestinal functions.
- Helps in production of hormones, enzymes and take part in many body functions.

Magnesium rich foods

- Fatty fishes: Salmon. Halibut. Mackerel.
- Nuts and seeds. pumpkin seeds.
- Fresh fruits. Bananas. Avocados.
- Whole grains: Wheat. Oat. Barley. Quinoa.
- Dark green leafy vegetables. Spinach.
- Legumes. Lentils. Black beans. Peas.
- Dark chocolates. Tofu.

Benefits of magnesium

- Magnesium acts as a co-factor in more than 300 enzyme system in the body that regulates
  - DNA and protein synthesis.
  - muscle and nerve function.
  - blood glucose and blood pressure regulation.
  - energy production in cells.
  - bone formation.
- Maintains healthy immune system, keeps the heartbeat steady, helps bones remain strong and helps adjust blood glucose levels.
- Boost exercise performance.
- Prevents depression.
- Anti-inflammatory effect.
- Low magnesium level cause
  - muscle weakness, fatigue.
  - muscle spasm and cramps.
  - numbness.
  - convulsions.
  - abnormal eye movements.

Potassium rich foods

- Dark green leafy vegetables. Spinach.
- Fish: Salmon. Perch.
- Beef. Sweet potato. Potato.
- Dry and fresh fruits: Orange. Apricot. Artichoke. Cantaloupe. Date. Raisine. Prunes. Banana. Orange. Avocado. Coconut water.
- Beans. Dried beans. Lentils. Beets. Parsnips. Tomato. Pea.
- Milk. Yogurt.

Benefits of potassium

- Proper nerve functions and muscle contraction.
- Maintains regular heartbeats.
- Transports nutrients into cells and waste products out of cells.
- Potassium helps to offset some of sodium's harmful effects on blood pressure.
- Maintains calcium level in blood.
- Potassium may help
  - manage blood pressure.
  - prevent stroke.
  - prevent kidney stones.
  - boost bone health.
  - manage blood glucose levels.
- Potassium deficiency may cause
  - high blood pressure.
  - kidney stones.
  - low calcium levels in the bones.
  - constipation.
  - fatigue, muscle weakness.
  - general feeling of being unwell or malaise.

Zinc rich foods

- Whole grains.
- Red meat. Poultry. Eggs. Oysters. Shellfish.
- Nuts and seeds.
- Dairy products: Milk. Cheese.
- Beans. Legumes. Lentils. Peas.

Benefits of Zinc.

- Boost-up immune system.
- Enhance wound healing.
- Improves metabolism and body function.
- Improves sense of taste and smell.
- Increase testosterone production and male sex vigour.

Vitamin A (retinol) rich foods

Only found in animal-sourced foods.

- Milk and milk products: Cheese. Butter.
- Oily fishes: Cod liver oil. Salmon. Tuna. Trout. Mackerel.
- Eggs.
- Beef liver. Lamb liver.
- *Carotenoid* containing foods: Body can produce vitamin A from carotenoids. They are found in plants:
  - Green leafy vegetables: Kale. Spinach. Lettuce. Turnip greens.
  - Colored fruits: Water melon. Tomato. Carrot. Papaya. Mango. Sweet potato. Apricot. Guava. Cantaloupe.

Benefits of vitamin A

- Maintains normal vision. Protects eyes from night blindness and age related decline of vision.
  - Supports bone, teeth and skin health.
  - Maintains a healthy immune system.
  - Promotes healthy growth and reproduction by gene transcription and protein formation.
  - May lower the risks of certain cancers.

Vitamin D rich foods

Sun is one of the best source of this nutrient. Spending time in sunlight is required.

Food sources are:

- Oily fishes: Salmon. Sardins. Tuna. Herring. Mackerel. Cod liver oil.
- Red meat. Cow and goat liver.
- Milk and dairy products: Yogurt. Cheese.
- Egg yolks (yellow part of egg).
- Fortified foods: Dairy products. Juices. Soy milk. Cereals. Margarine.
- Mushrooms.
- Vegetables: Beans. Dark green leafy vegetables. Okra.

Benefits of vitamin D

- Builds and maintains strong bones and teeth.
- Supports proper functioning of immune system, brain and nervous system.
- Supports lung and heart functions.
- Regulates insulin secretion and manage diabetes.
- May help in supporting cognitive health. Improves mood and reduces depression.
- Benefits sexual health in man.

Vitamin E rich foods

- Wheat germ oil.
- Plant oils: Sunflower. Safflower. Soya. Olive oil. Corn oil.
- Nuts and seeds: Sunflower. Safflower. Almonds and other nuts. Pumpkin seeds. Peanut butter.
- Dark leafy green vegetables. Avocado.
- Fishes.

Benefits of vitamin E

- It is an anti-oxident.
- Supports immune function.
- Prevents inflammation and coronary heart diseases.
- Boosts-up fertility especially in women.
- Promotes eye health.
- Delay Alzheimer's disease.

Vitamin K rich foods

- Green leafy vegetables.
- Fish. Meat. Egg. Beef and lamb liver.
- Fruits: Berries. Kiwi. Avocado. Fig. Tomato. Dried plum.

Benefits of vitamin K.

- Essential for healthy blood clotting function.
- Regulates blood calcium level and bone formation.
- Improves high blood pressure and body circulation.
- Improves memory function of brain.
- Lowers the risk of stroke.

BODY PAIN AND PAIN RELIEF

Vitamin C rich foods

- Citrus fruits: Orange. Kiwifruit. Lemon. Grape fruit. Guava. Papaya.
- All berries.
- Peppers: Green and red peppers. Bell peppers.
- Cruciferous vegetables: Broccoli. Cauliflower. Cabbage. Brussels sprouts.
- Dark leafy green vegetables.
- Potatoes. Peas. Tomatoes.
- Cantaloupe. Rock melon. Sweet melon. Spanspek.

Vitamin C and B-vitamins are reduced on cooking. Vitamin C is destroyed by light.

Benefits of vitamin C

- It is a powerful anti-oxidant.
- Necessary for growth, development and repair of all body tissue.
- Essential for wound healing.
- Prevents common cold.
- Maintenence of health of bones, teeth, and cartilage.
- Helps absorption of iron and selenium.
- Boosts immunity.
- Manage high blood pressure and lowers heart disease.
- Reduces the risk of chronic disease.
- Memory boost-up in older age group and prevention of dementia.

Vitamin B rich foods

- Milk. Cheese.
- Meat: Red meat. Liver. Kidney. Poultry. Eggs.
- Fishes. Shellfish.
- Dark leafy green vegetables. Spinach. Kale. Beets. Avocados. Wheat germ.
- Whole grains and cereals. Potatoes. Soy products.
- All beans. All nuts and seeds.
- Citrus fruits. Banana. water melon.
- Molasses. Yeast and nutritional yeast.

Benefits of vitamin B-complex.

- Support and promote cell health and function.
- Heart function improves.
- Enhance growth of blood forming cells.
- Carbohydrate metabolism improves.
- Enzyme and hormone production improves.
- Improves energy levels of the body.
- Improvement of eye sights.
- Healthy brain and nerve functions.
- Improves appetite and digestive function.
- Prevents infection.
- Improves muscle tone, strength and flexibility.
- Erectile dysfunction improves.
- Prevention of fetal birth defects.
- Reduction of pregnancy complications.

Prebiotic foods

Prebiotics are fibers and natural sugars that stimulate the good bacteria in the gut. These foods include:

- Whole grains. Soybeans. Almond.
- Garlic. Onion. Chicory root.
- Banana. Asparagus. Leeks.
- Chick pea. Dandelion greens.

Probiotic foods

Probiotics are live bacteria and yeasts that are good for health. Probiotics are called good or helpful bacteria because they help to keep the gut healthy. They help in digestive health, immune function and in weight loss. Foods with probiotics include:

- Yogurt: made from goat or cow's milk.
- Kefir: made from kefir grains.
- Sauerkraut: made from cabbage.
- Tempeh: fermented soybean product.
- Kimchi.

BODY PAIN AND PAIN RELIEF

Anti-oxident rich foods

- All berries.
- Dark green leafy vegetables. Red cabbage. Carrot. Broccoli.
- Sweet potato. Asparagus. Squash. Pumpkin. Artichokes.
- Whole grains. Oatmeal. Beans. Nuts.
- Fishes.
- Beet roots. Radish. Pecans.
- Green tea. Yogurt.
- Vitamin C containing foods. chart.
- Dark chocolate. Avocado.
- Body makes glutathione.

Functions of anti-oxidents.

- Anti-oxidents stabilize free radicals and scavanges free radicles from the body. Free radicles damage normal and aged cells in the body. Free radicals can trigger inflammation and damage cells.
- Reduce cell damage.
- Retards aging process.
- Increases good HDL cholesterol.
- Reduce the risk of heart disease.
- Reduces joint inflammation.
- Reduce the risk of certain cancers like prostate cancers.
- Lower the incidence of eye lens degeneration.
- Delay the onset of Alzheimer's disease and Parkinson's disease.

Omega-3 fatty acid rich foods

- Fish: cold water fatty fish: salmon. mackerel. sardines. cod liver oil. tuna. herring. anchovies. caviar. trout. halibut.
- Seafood: algal oil. Oyster.
- Nuts and seeds: flaxseed, chiaseed, hempseed, pumpkin seed, Walnut.
- Plant oils: flaxseed oil, soybean oil, canola oil, perilla oil.
- Dark green leafy vegetables. Brussels sprouts.

Functions of omega-3 fatty acids.

- Reduce LDL and other bad fats.
- Slow the development of plaque and clot in the blood vessels.
- Reduce the chance of abnormal heart rhythm.
- Reduce the likelihood of heart attack and stroke.

- Reduce the chance of sudden cardiac death in people with heart disease.
- Beneficial in high blood pressure.
- Fights inflammation in the body.
- Improve bone and joint health.
- Improve eye and skin health.
- Improve sleep.
- Reduce symptoms of metabolic syndrome.
- Alleviate menstrual pain.
- Reduce asthma in children.
- Improve mental disorder.
- Promote brain health in infant.
- Reduce the symptoms of attention deficit hyperactivity disorder (ADHD) in children.
- Prevent cancer.

Foods rich in trans-fatty acids (bad fats for heart)

- Backery foods: cakes, cookies, pies, biscuits, rolls, patty, pastry, ladoo.
- Fried foods: French fries, doughnuts, fried chicken, puff.
- Non-dairy coffee creamer.
- Stick margarine, Vanaspati, coconut oil.
- Frozen pizza, Microwave popcorn.

Foods rich in omega-6 fatty acids

- Corn. Sunflower and safflower.
- Soybeans. Peanut. Nuts and seeds.
- Mayonnaise. Meat, fish, poultry, eggs.
- Salad dressings.

Omega-3 fatty acids are more beneficial than omega-6 fatty acids.

Foods rich in histamine

- Alcohol and other fermented beverages and foods.
- Shellfish. Dairy products. Yogurt. Processed and smoked meat and foods.
- Eggplant. Spinach. Dried fruits.

Benefits of walking

- Maintains healthy body weight.
- Prevents back, neck and hip pain.
- Promotes better balance and stability to the spine.
- Reduces the risks of falling and injury.
- Strengthens abdominal, back, leg and buttock muscles.
- Improves walking speed, distence and stride.
- Increases energy levels of the body.
- Improves heart function and blood circulation.
- Breathing functions improves and become easy.
- Makes stronger bones and muscles.
- Body fat reduced.
- Improves muscles and joints functions.
- Lose body weight.
- Improves digestive function.
- Prevents heart disease, stroke, high blood pressure, some cancer and type 2 diabetes.
- Reduces mental stress and anxiety.
- Ensure sound sleep.
- Mood stabilization and improvement.
- Longer life span.

Benefits of regular physical activities and exercises

- Improve blood supply to whole body tissue.
- Improve brain function and memory.
- Improve quality of sleep.
- Healthy body weight management.
- Reduce feeling of anxiety and depression.
- Improve heart health and blood pressure.

Breathing exercise

Slow but deep inhalation and exhalation is breathing exercise.

Method:

- Sit or lie flat in a comfortable position.
- One hand is put on the belly below the ribs and the other hand is on the chest.

- Inhale slowly and deeply through the nose. Shoulder and body should be kept relaxed.
- At the end of breath in, the air in the lungs should be holded for 2-3 seconds before breathing out.
- Exhale slowly through the pursed lips as if whistling. Jaws are kept relaxed.
- Do this for several minutes/3-10 times.

Benefits of deep breathing exercises:

- Improves blood flow in the body.
- Reduce stress level in the body.
- Reduce anxiety and depression.
- Relaxes mind and body.
- Reduce fatigueness.
- Lower blood pressure and heart rate.
- Improves digestion.
- Improve diabetic symptoms.
- Natural pain killer. Chronic body pain is relieved.
- Detoxifies the body.
- Reduce inflammation in the body.

Benefits of swimming

- It is the best non-weight bearing exercise.
- It is a relaxing and peaceful form of exertcise.
- Improves heart function and muscle strength.
- Improves joint flexibility and movedment.
- Improves coordination,balance and posture.
- Maintains healthy weight,healthy heart and lungs.
- Reduce body fat and weight.

Benefits of warm pool swimming

- Pool temperature should be between 78-86°F.
- Relaxes muscles and joints.
- Reduce joint inflammation.
- Relieves pain in joints.
- Improves blood circulation and breathing.
- Relieves mental stress.

BODY PAIN AND PAIN RELIEF

Benefits of steam bath
- Improves blood circulation and reduces body pain.
- Improves skin circulation and skin texture.
- Burns calories and maintain healthy body weight.
- Improves flexibility of stiff joints.
- Improves muscle and joint functions.
- Reduces mental stress and anxiety.

Benefits of jogging and running
- Strengthen muscles.
- Build strong bones.
- Improves heart function and blood circulation.
- Reduce weight and maintain a healthy body weight.

Hot compression

Hot compression is best for long standing (chronic) pain. It helps in dilation of blood vessels and thus blood supply to the area is increased. The ultimate result is proper distribution of nutrients to the cells and helps to flush out the toxins from the body. Heat therapy should be applied under supervision.

Benefits of hot compression:

- Relieves pain and inflammation.
- Muscles are relaxed and pain is relieved.
- Flushes toxins from the body and relieves pain.
- Relieves chronic joint pain.
- Improves joint flexibility.
- Wound healing is accelerated.

Cold compression

Cold compression is best for short term (acute) pain. It may be applied within 48 hours after an injury. Cold compression works by constricting the surrounding blood vessels and thus reduces swelling and inflammation and thus relieves pain. Patient also becomes less sensitive to pain due to reduction of nerve activity. Cold compression should be applied under supervision.

Benefits of cold compression:

- Sooth the injured muscles, joints and other tissues.
- General pain relief by decreasing nerve activity.

- Stops bleeding within tissues and organs.

Uses:

- Sprain and strain of joints, muscles, ligaments and tendons.
- Imflammation and pain.
- Inflammation of joints (arthritis)
- Knee sprain (Runner's knee).
- Inflammation of tendons (Tendonitis).
- Acute low back pain.
- After operation in a joint.

Massage therapy

Massage is a type of physiotherapy where rubbing, pressing and manipulations are done by a trained physiotherapist with expert hands. Muscles, tendons, ligaments and skin are massaged. The tissues are rubbed, tapped, stroked and kneaded. Massage therapy may help people to relax, relieve stress and pain and improve circulation. Proper massage therapy may also lower blood pressure.

Benefits of massage therapy:

- Improves blood supply to the area.
- Reduces muscle tension and spasm and causes muscle relaxation. Reduces muscle stiffness.
- Reduce inflammation.
- Improves joint mobility and flexibility.
- Soft tissue injury recovers better.
- Reduces stress and pain in an area.
- Lowers heart rate and blood pressure.
- Reduces stress and anxiety.
- Improves skin tone.

Uses.

- Low back pain.Upper back and neck pain.
- Headache.Muscle pain.
- Soft tissue sprain and strain.
- Sports injury.

Firm mattress

A firm mattress is firm to feel. It should not feel like a plank of wood or doesn't have a soft or, sinking feeling. Firm mattress gives a sturdy support to the spine and the body as a whole. It will hold the body in a neutral position.

Benefits of firm mattress:

- Prevents collapsing and sagging of lower back.
- Weight of the body is distributed evenly on the mattress, so, no one part of the body bears the stress of pressure.
- Muscles are less strained, and circulation is improved.
- Supports the spine firmly and eliminate back pain.

Benefits of getting enough sleep

- Improves mood. Ensures healthy body and mind.
- Reduction of stress and anxiety.
- Improves vital functions of body.
- Clear thinking and sound working output.
- Boost-up immunity of the body.
- Improves heart functions, work output, memory and learning.
- Prevents frequent illness.
- Body metabolism improves, thus improving general health condition. Healthy body weight is maintained.

High glycemic index foods (bad for diabetic patients)

- whole wheat. White wheat bread. White rice.
- Refined sugar. Honey. Cakes. Cookies. Sweet backary items.
- Corn flakes. Pop corn. Breakfast cereals. Instant pasta.
- Potatoes. Chips and rice crackers.
- Fruits: watermelon. pineapple. pumpkin.
- Dried fruits: Dates. Raisins. Cranberries.
- Pear. Pear juice.
- Ice cream. Rice milk.

Low glycemic index foods (relatively good for diabetic patients)

- Oatmeal. Barley. Rolled oats. Steel-cut oats.
- Non-starchy vegetables. Green vegetables. Sweet potatoes. Egg plant. Cauliflower. Brussels sprouts. Broccoli. Zucchini. Swiss chard.

- Kidney beans. Chick peas. Lentils. Pea nuts. Peas. Carrots.
- Milk. Skim milk. Plain yogurt. Full fat yogurt. Cheese. Butter. Cream.
- Most fruits. Apple. Berries. Avocado. Olives. Kiwis. Apricots.
- Low carbohydrate and non-carbohydrate foods.
    - Lean meat. Egg. Beef. Lamb. Chicken.
    - Fish: most of fishes.
    - Seafoods.
    - Leafy green vegetables: see names.
    - Nuts, seeds, beans. Nut butter. Almond. Wallnut. Peanut. Chia seeds. Flax seeds. Sunflower seeds. Pistachios. Pumpkin seeds.
    - Oils. Olive oil. Coconut oil. Rapseed oil.
    - Spices. Onion. Garlic. Bell pepper.
    - Tomato. Mushrooms. Asparagus. Lemon.
- Sugar free beverages: Plain water. Coffee. Tea. Carbonated water.
- Dark chocolates.

Complex carbohydrates (relatively good for diabetics).

- Whole-wheat breads, Brown rice. Quinoa.
- Oatmeal, corn.
- Peas, beans. Lentils.
- Green and colored leafy vegetables.
- Starchy vegetables. chart.

Starchy vegetables (relatively bad for diabetic patients).

- White potatoes, Sweet potatoes, Beets, Carrots.
- Corn, Peas, Squash, Pumpkin, Turnips.

Non-starchy vegetables (relatively good for diabetic patients).

- Leafy green vegetables, Cabbage, Cauliflower, Kale.
- Baby corn, Bamboo shoots, Cucumber, Spinach.
- Beans, Broccoli, Mushrooms, Asparagus, Artichoke.
- Eggplant, Celery, Onion, Peepers.

Benefits of green tea

- Lower total cholesterol, LDL and triglycerides.
- Better control of blood pressure.
- Increases fat burning and lose weight.
- Prevent cell damage and reduce inflammation.
- Improve insulin sensitivity and diabetes is improved.

- Anti-oxident action.
- Improve brain function.
- Reduced risk of cancer.
- Helps to live longer.

Benefits of garlic

- Regulates blood glucose and reduces certain complications of diabetes.
- Lowers LDL (bad fat).
- Inhibit build-up of plaque in the blood vessels and improve circulation and lowers blood pressure. Prevent heart disease.
- Boost-up immunity and Fights infection.
- Acts as powerful anti-oxident and anti-inflammatory agent.

Prevents cellular transformation and cellular mutation and thus reduces risks of cancer.

Glossary

Abdomen: is also called the 'belly' or 'tummy' and is the part of the body between the chest and the pelvis.

Acute: severe and sudden in onset.

Chronic: of long duration. Continuing or occurring again and again for a long time.

Degeneration: is the deterioration and loss of function in the cells of a tissue or organ.

Fascia: fascia is a thin sheet of fibrous tissue that covers and holds different tissues and organs.

Fibrous tissue: It is composed of closely woven small fibers. They form a network or adhere together to form tendon, ligament, fascia etc.

Groin: the depression between the thigh and trunk. This area is also called as the inguinal region.

Hormone: hormone is a secretion of the ductless gland in the body. They are carried by blood to the target organs and produce actions.

Infection: a disease caused by microorganisms, like bacteria, virus, fungus etc.

Inflammation: is a localised physical condition in which a part of the body becomes reddened, swollen, hot and often painful, especially as a reaction to injury or infection.

Ligament: ligament is the fibrous tissue like rope, that ties bone to other bone. They are most abundant within and around joints.

Loin: loin is the part of the body at the lower part of the back and sides between the ribs and the hip.

Membrane: a thin layer of cells acting as a boundary, lining or partition of tissue or organ.

Musculoskeletal: related to muscles and skeleton.

Pelvis: It is a large bony structure formed by two hip bones and lower part of spine. Two lower limbs are connected with it by hip joints.

Symptom: any change in the body or its functions as perceived by the patient. (Taber).

Tendon: tendon is rope like fibrous tissue which is firmly connected to muscle fibers at one end and to the bone at the other end. Tendon transmits the mechanical force of muscle contraction to the bone.

Ulcer: is an open sore on an external or internal surface of the body, and is caused by a break or infection in the skin or other membrane that fails to heal.

References

Sources of informations:

- Apley's System of orthopaedics & fractures.
- Complete Family nutrition by DK publishing.
- Food & nutrition what everyone needs to know.
- Food nutrition & wellness student edition.
- Stretching to stay Young - Jessica.
- The anatomy of stretching - Brad walker.
- Restorative Yoga for beginners.
- Yoga for men.
- Boundless – Ben Greenfield.
- Stretching therapy.
- Therapeutic Exercise-Foundations and Techniques-Carolyn Kisner, Borstad, Colby.
- Joint structure and function-Levangie, Norkin.
- Davidson's Principles & Practice of Medicine.
- Park's text book of Preventive and Social Medicine.
- DC Dutta's textbook of Gynaecology.
- Tuberculosis of the skeletal system – S M Tuli.
- Bailey & Love's short practice of Surgery.
- Obstetrics by Ten Teachers.
- Ganong's Review of medical physiology.
- Guyton and Hall Textbook of Medical physiology.
- Gray's Anatomy – Elsevier.

www.ingramcontent.com/pod-product-compliance
Lightning Source LLC
Chambersburg PA
CBHW052341220526
45465CB00003BA/907